A fellow traveler on the road to health & happiness

Milano

skinny is
overrated

The Real Woman's Guide to

Health and Happiness at

Any Size

Danielle Milano, MD

Synergy Books

Skinny Is Overrated: The Real Woman's Guide to Health and Happiness at Any Size
Published by Synergy Books
P.O. Box 30071
Austin, Texas 78755

For more information about our books, please write us, e-mail us at info@synergybooks.net, or visit our web site at www.synergybooks.net.

Publisher's Cataloging-in-Publication
(Provided by Quality Books, Inc.)

Milano, Danielle.
    Skinny is overrated : the real woman's guide to
health and happiness at any size / Danielle Milano.
    p. cm.
    Includes bibliographical references and index.
    LCCN 2009937950
    ISBN-13: 978-0-9842358-3-4
    ISBN-10: 0-9842358-3-3

    1. Women--Health and hygiene. 2. Overweight women.
3. Nutrition. 4. Exercise for women.   I. Title.

RA778.M55 2010   613'.04244
                            QBI09-600193

As with any diet and exercise plan, check with your physician before embarking on this program. It is especially important to check with your physician if you are diabetic, if you are very overweight or out of shape, if heart disease runs in your family, or if you smoke. This is not an all-inclusive list; there are many other health conditions that should be addressed before you start an exercise plan. True, exercise helps people live longer, healthier lives, but be safe. Schedule an appointment with your physician before you start any diet and exercise program.

Front cover design by Priyanka Kodikal.

10 9 8 7 6 5 4 3 2 1

To the memory of my mother, an amazing cook, who was committed to keeping her family healthy through nutritious food. She was ahead of her time.

Table of Contents

Introduction

Welcome to East Harlem, "El Barrio." Located in upper Manhattan, it's a lively immigrant neighborhood. In other words, it's a neighborhood of the poor.

In 1999, I came to the Boriken Clinic in El Barrio to care for HIV patients, but patients with diabetes quickly started to fill my waiting room. One by one, little by little, these diabetic patients took over my practice. More out of control than HIV, obesity and diabetes are decimating my patients, the people of El Barrio, and Americans all over the country.

We do not need fancy studies to see why this is happening. You can find the answer if you simply walk the four blocks from the subway station to the clinic where I work. On your walk, you would pass scores of people rushing to work, to school, or just hanging out on the corner with friends. As you pass people on that four-block walk, you would notice that something is wrong. Why are so many middle-aged people in wheelchairs and young adults using canes? Why do so many people, young and old, have rotten teeth? Why don't the teenagers have the glow you see in kids when they are young, healthy, and athletic? And finally, why is everyone so *big*?

The answer lies in the restaurants you pass along the way. You could grab a hamburger and fries, or even donuts and ice cream, for lunch. If you're in the mood for Spanish food, there is a "cuchifrito" selling roast pork and fried plantains on every corner. Feel like fried chicken? Just walk half a block the other way. If money is tight, there are plenty of pizza parlors, and don't forget the dollar menu at McDonald's. If you want a salad, you're out of luck.

What does this have to do with diabetes? Everything! Unhealthy eating habits, along with lack of exercise, lead to obesity, which then leads to diabetes. When people have diabetes, they simply don't feel good. Their energy levels are low. People turn to fast food because grocery shopping and cooking take work. The children eat the same unhealthy foods as their parents, which perpetuates the vicious cycle of obesity and diabetes through generations.

Where should one begin the quest to get healthy? There is so much information on health and dieting out there; it's confusing. People simply don't know how to eat healthy anymore. Patients ask me all the time to tell them what to eat. Unfortunately, you cannot squeeze a lifetime of learning into the few minutes we have during an appointment. To make sure everyone has access to practical information, I have spent the last three years writing this book.

This book is for my patients who keep begging, "Tell me what to eat." Realize, though, that you need to focus on health, not on weight. Since most of my patients are women, this book is geared toward them. Weight seems to be more of an issue for women than men, thanks to pressure from magazines to be thin and beautiful. Fortunately, my patients are not obsessed with being thin, but they do need to lose some weight. Even a little bit of weight loss improves health for those who are overweight or obese. But weight is not the only factor that determines health; fitness is far more important.

Fitness is the result of exercise, and the most important lifestyle change you can make is to start exercising. Study after study has shown that exercise prevents diseases like diabetes and hypertension. People who exercise vigorously, like runners, live longer, healthier lives than their couch-potato cousins. If running is out of the question, even walking is enough to maintain fitness and health.

The next hurdle for many is to stop drinking soda. Extra calories from soda and sweets are stored in the belly as fat. This belly fat puts people at high risk for developing diabetes, hypertension, heart attacks, and strokes.

Diet is the last step. This book will not give you a list of what to eat every day. Instead, it's an education on the components of the Mediterranean diet interpreted for present-day America, so people can make it their own. The Mediterranean diet has been shown over and over again to be a healthy diet. Diabetics' blood sugar improves, blood pressure goes down, and people live longer. Experts have different opinions as to the magic ingredient of the Mediterranean diet. Is it the red wine, the olive oil, or the omega-3 oils in fish? In my opinion, the magic is in the mighty vegetable. Vegetables are vital, and because people don't know how to cook fresh vegetables in a tasty way, there are recipes and instructions on cooking techniques at the end of this book.

Other traditional diets, not just the Mediterranean diet, are healthy as well. If your ancestors came from Central America, South America, Africa, Asia, or the Caribbean, chances are they lived a healthy lifestyle that included plenty of exercise and a diet full of vegetables. Perhaps we should look back to our roots and incorporate those healthy aspects of the traditional lifestyle of our ancestors into our own lives.

The concept of a low-fat diet needs to be put to rest. Low-fat diets don't work and are especially bad for diabetics. Fats are important for health, but they must be healthy fats from nuts, fish, and olive oil. Trans fats need to be avoided completely.

Since everyone has to start somewhere, I give an overview of motivation and goal setting. Wanting to be healthy isn't enough. People need to set goals and see the ways they sabotage themselves.

I also cover other components of a healthy lifestyle: vitamin D, calcium, and antioxidants. Since food is expensive, don't waste your money on supplements and gym memberships. Spend that money on fresh fruits and vegetables.

Health is about changing your lifestyle through physical activity and plenty of satisfying food. It is about changing the way you approach life, feeling better about yourself, and living life to its fullest. You deserve to be happy, healthy, vital, and fulfilled. If you are obese or out of shape, you will never achieve the full extent of greatness of which you are capable.

Chapter One

If You Put a Bulldog on a Diet, You Don't End Up with a Greyhound

I t's obvious. All the diets in the world could never turn a bull-dog into a greyhound, and it's no different for people. If you have ever dieted, you know how hard it is to lose weight and keep it off, but why? Let's put it into perspective by using some examples.

The first example looks at people who are naturally thin. Although you might be jealous, it's just as difficult for a thin person to gain weight as it is for an obese person to lose it. A few years back, obesity researchers did an experiment with men who were naturally thin.[1] The men volunteered to gain weight, and because the "volunteers" were in prison, the number of calories eaten could be measured carefully. Over the course of six months, the group ate a lot. All of the men gained quite a bit of weight; some gained as much as fifty pounds. The experiment ended, and the volunteers went back to their old eating habits. The men did not "go on a diet." They ate when they were hungry and stopped when they were satisfied. Each man lost every pound gained. It took a few

---

1. E. A. Sims, "Experimental Obesity, Dietary-Induced Thermogenesis, and Their Clinical Implications," *Clinics in Endocrinology and Metabolism* 5, no. 2 (1976): 377–395.

months, but every volunteer ended up back at his starting weight. These naturally thin men gravitated back to their original weight by eating to the level of their hunger.

Another story makes this point in a slightly different way. Years ago, adoption agencies would separate twins. Fortunately, this is no longer practiced in the United States, but back then, one baby would go to one set of parents and the other twin would go to another. One such set of twin girls found each other many years later as adults. One twin had exercised and dieted constantly throughout the years. The other twin had eaten whatever she wanted and never followed an exercise regimen. After all those years of diet and exercise, the dieting twin only weighed five pounds less than her sister.

A number of studies, called *twin studies*, have been done to look at whether genetics or your home life is more important in determining weight. This is called *nature versus nurture*. *Nature* refers to the genes you inherited from your parents. *Nurture* refers to the foods you ate, the schools you attended, and everything else that goes on in your life.

Since identical twins have the same genes, if the twins grew up in separate households, researchers could look at the impact of the environment, like food, exercise, and social issues, on weight. By using twin studies, some obesity researchers estimate that as much as 70 percent of our weight is determined by our genetic makeup. Just as the thin men easily lost fifty pounds, the overweight and the obese will easily gain back all of the weight lost from dieting. We all gravitate to a weight determined by our genes. People who are naturally heavy are hungry after losing weight through dieting. Levels of hunger hormones, i.e., hormones telling us to eat, are actually higher after a diet. Is it any wonder dieters gain back all of the weight they worked so hard to lose?

Yet, separated twins could grow up in similar environments, eating the same type of foods and getting the nearly the same amount of exercise, which would make it difficult to tell how much of their weight was a result of their genes and how much was their environment. As such, researchers decided to look at another group, the Pima Indians. About one thousand years ago, some of the Pima Indian tribe migrated to the United States, while others stayed in Mexico. Although not twins, they are very closely related. A Pima woman living in Mexico weighs on average fifty pounds less than a Pima woman living in Arizona and has a far lower risk of developing diabetes. The Pima Indians living the traditional lifestyle in Mexico work hard, very hard, to put food on the table. They grow vegetables in the backyard without fancy tractors and walk miles every day. They don't eat much processed foods, or as much food in general, as we do in the United States. When obesity researchers consider the Pima Indians, they are led to believe that maybe family genes only contribute to 30 percent of our weight.

Whether it's 30 percent or 70 percent, don't give up! There is hope. Remember that the goal is to live a long, healthy, active life. One does not need to be thin to be fit and healthy.

Chapter Two

Identify with Your Heritage

ike the Pima, most of us can trace our ancestry to another country, or continent. We have parents, grandparents, or great-grandparents who moved to America from another country. While some of us arrived recently, others have forefathers who have lived in America for hundreds of years. No matter how far back you can trace your ancestry, think back to how your relatives lived and how they ate in the past. If you have any questions about the traditional foods of your ancestors, you could browse the cookbook aisles at your local bookstore, or look on the Internet. There are thousands of cookbooks from all over the globe.

Most of us identify strongly with our heritage, not through the language or the music, but through the food. This book is based on a Mediterranean diet, which may not appeal to you. Look back, then, at your own heritage for ideas. Chances are your ancestors ate a healthier diet than you do now.

Certainly, some cultures are not known for their healthy foods; British and Eastern European cultures spring to mind. My Jewish friends make fun of their childhood meals. The only vegetable served was cabbage, with the exception of canned peas and carrots dished up as a special treat.

But if you or your ancestors are from Central America, South America, Asia, Africa, or certain areas of Europe, chances are your relatives lived a healthier lifestyle than you do now. There is a new book out called *The Blue Zones: Lessons for Living Longer from the People Who've Lived the Longest*. As part of a large research study, the author traveled around the world to places where people are more likely to live to be one hundred years old. These Blue Zones are in far-flung places: Okinawa, Japan; the island of Sardinia off the coast of Italy; Costa Rica; and a community of Seventh-day Adventists in Lima Linda, California. Obviously, shepherds in Sardinia are not eating tofu, and the Seventh-day Adventists are not drinking red wine since they abstain from alcohol completely. The diets may not seem similar, but in broad brushstrokes, there are similarities in the lifestyles of these four groups of people from four different continents. All four groups eat plenty of vegetables every day, and all continue to be physically active well into old age.

Look back to your roots. Incorporate the healthy aspects of that diet and lifestyle. No matter where your predecessors are from, I am certain that soda, fast food, and processed foods were not part of the daily diet. Meals were always homemade. Most likely, fruits and vegetables, beans, and legumes predominated. In Italy, especially during the winter, dinner was often a rich soup made with beans and pasta, or lentils and barley. Meat was a luxury, and when available, the portions served were small when compared to American standards. You wouldn't find sixteen-ounce charbroiled sirloin steaks on the menu. That much steak would serve a family of four, with the rest of their dinner plates piled with vegetables.

People from islands and coastal regions ate fish. Ceviche, raw seafood "cooked" in lime juice, continues to be a South American specialty. But if your ancestors were from the mountains, fish was even more of a luxury than meat. For example, my grandmother was from a mountainous region in southern Italy. Dried salt cod was the only fish I ever learned to cook from her. On the other hand, a friend of mine is of Portuguese descent. Your mouth waters when she talks about the fish stews of her childhood. Still, even people from coastal regions didn't eat fish every day. Her mom was just as likely to serve a bean soup as a fish stew. She would use black beans, white beans, red beans, speckled beans, and beans my friend can't identify anymore.

In addition to bean soups, each Mediterranean culture has a variation of soups made with green leafy vegetables. You may have seen "wedding" soup on the menu at some Italian restaurants, although I have never once seen it served at any of my relatives' weddings. It's soup made with either escarole or dandelion greens, and we had it every year at Christmas. We weren't eating soup for dinner during the summer, but no matter the time of the year, there was always a green leafy vegetable on the table.

Meals were never washed down with soda. If you're of Chinese or Japanese descent, you drank tea. If you're Greek, Italian, French, or Portuguese, you drank red wine with dinner, although teas made with chamomile or other local dried herbs were enjoyed for their health benefits.

As for dessert, no matter where your ancestors are from, it was never a double fudge sundae. Dessert would be fruits in season. There is nothing as delicious as a big bowl of fresh grapes. Researchers are finding that there is a special compound in grapes that may help people live longer. If your ancestors were lucky enough to be from a sunny climate, they had fruits all year round.

And consider the women of France: they stay slim through middle age. Why? They never go back for second helpings. They practiced portion control long before it became a buzzword in nutrition circles.

Most of you know what you need to do: replace some or most of your meat-based meals with bean dishes or fish stews. Replace your sugary desserts with fruit. Stop drinking soda. Stop eating processed foods. Eat loads more vegetables. Limit your portion size.

Don't fall for all the hype about dieting you hear on the news and from the media. If you get back to your roots, it will be easy for you to change your lifestyle back into a healthy one.

Chapter Three

Get Motivated!

Are you overweight, obese, very obese? Check the chart below to find out. Find your height and see if your weight falls into the category of obesity. BMI refers to Body Mass Index. It's an easy measurement used by physicians to rate whether someone is underweight, of normal weight, overweight, obese, or very obese.

Height (feet and inches)	Overweight: BMI 25–30	Obese: BMI 30–40
5'0"	125–150 pounds	155–205 pounds
5'1"	130–155 pounds	160–212 pounds
5'2"	135–160 pounds	165–219 pounds
5'3"	140–165 pounds	170–226 pounds
5'4"	145–170 pounds	175–233 pounds
5'5"	150–175 pounds	180–241 pounds
5'6"	155–180 pounds	185–249 pounds
5'7"	160–185 pounds	190–256 pounds
5'8"	165–190 pounds	195–264 pounds
5'9"	170–195 pound	200–272 pounds
5'10"	175–200 pounds	210–280 pounds
5'11"	180–205 pounds	215–288 pounds

If your weight is off the chart, you're considered very obese.

When an overweight or obese patient comes into the clinic to see me, I pull out my little Body Mass Index calculator from the Department of Health. The mathematical formula to calculate BMI is your weight (in kilograms) divided by your height (in meters) squared. That's why we use charts and calculators that do the math for us.

Consider this young woman. At five feet four inches tall and 250 pounds, she has a BMI of forty-three, which is considered very obese. She asked me what she should weigh, and with my trusty little calculator, I told her the Department of Health says she should weigh 124 pounds. We both had a laugh because that is such an unreasonable number. First of all, she doesn't want to weigh 124 pounds. Second of all, telling someone to lose 126 pounds is such an enormous feat that I might as well tell her to go out and become an astronaut.

The point is to *forget about the BMI chart*. Don't worry about what the Department of Health wants you to weigh. There are more important questions: Can you walk up and down a flight of stairs? If there were a fire in your building, how many firemen would it take to carry you out? If it would take more than one fireman to save you (all right, two at the most), it's time to take action! Let's get motivated and do something about it!

For too long, the medical profession has focused on the negatives. We know all of the terrible things that can happen to you if you remain obese and don't exercise: diabetes, strokes, hypertension, knee replacements, heart attacks, and kidney failure. Forget all that negativity. Focus on the great things that would happen to you if you got just below that BMI of thirty. If you are starting out at five feet four inches and 250 pounds but slimmed down to 165 pounds by exercising and eating plenty of healthy food, you may not be skinny, but you would be healthy.

There's even more good news. In one large epidemiological study, the people who were overweight lived longer than the people who were underweight, obese, or even of an ideal weight.[1] Well, we know that people who are obese die of heart attacks, strokes, and diabetes; and people who are underweight die of lung disease. But why would people who are overweight live longer than people who are considered of normal or "ideal" weight? No one knows, and quite a few scientists are scratching their heads thinking about it. Realize that there are other studies in which people with an ideal body weight lived longer than the overweight. Nevertheless, this one epidemiological study gives us hope. We can be overweight but still live long and healthy lives.

A woman who is five feet three inches is considered to have an ideal body weight if she weighs between 105 and 142 pounds. That same woman is considered *overweight* if she weighs between 142 and 165 pounds. When I say that overweight people live longer, I'm not talking about 100 pounds overweight. I'm talking specifically about just a few pounds. I'm talking about the overweight category on the BMI chart. A five-feet-three-inch woman who weighs more than 165 pounds is pushing the envelope if she tells you that she keeps the extra weight on so she can live longer. But to understand this, you do not need complicated research articles from prestigious medical journals stating the obvious. All you need to do is look at someone to know if that person is healthy, whether she is thin or packing a few extra pounds.

If you're obese and need to get down to the category of overweight, the road to turning your life around starts with a little inward reflection: Do you rationalize overeating? Do you make excuses for avoiding exercise? Do you buy potato chips and ice cream "for the kids" and then eat them yourself? I've heard some of the most outlandish excuses from my patients. It may be easier to recognize your own problem by seeing it in someone else.

See if you fit into one of these typical categories:

---

1. K. M. Flegal and others, "Cause-Specific Excess Deaths Associated with Underweight, Overweight, and Obesity," *Journal of the American Medical Association* 298, no. 17 (2007): 2028–2037.

The Slave

There are so many women who say they cannot eat healthy because it's too much trouble to cook one meal for themselves and a different meal for the family! It's health food, not torture food. Let the family eat healthy too.

If you're overweight, chances are your children are overweight too. Even if you're the only one in the family who is overweight, everyone in the family should be eating healthy. If they don't like it, they can cook for themselves. You are the boss; you are not a slave.

Plus, don't you want your children to eat healthy? They need essential fatty acids, vitamins, and minerals for their developing bodies. You know that you should not be eating potato chips because they are not good for you, but it's *okay* for the kids to eat them? Does this make any sense? Chips aren't any better for your children than they are for you.

The Self-Medicator

How about the women who eat because they are nervous or depressed? When did potato chips and ice cream become a cure for anxiety and depression? Think about this for a minute. You can look at alcoholics objectively and realize how ridiculous it is when they say that they drink because they are nervous or depressed. Having a drink makes them feel better, they say. To a nondrinker, looking in from the outside, it's obvious that having a drink is only making the problem worse.

It's the same with overeating. You need to realize you have a problem and deal with it. In twelve-step programs, they tell people who want to have a drink to HALT, which stands for Hungry, Angry, Lonely, or Thirsty. If someone feels she is going to relapse, she needs to take a moment to sort out her feelings and ask herself if she is hungry, angry, lonely, or thirsty. I've expanded it a bit to HHAALTT. Do you overeat because you are hurt, hungry, angry, anxious, lonely, tired, or thirsty? Add more to the list if you want.

Make up your own: BORFED (Bored, Frustrated, Depressed). Think about it before you overeat.

I call this "eating your emotions." Are you eating your emotions instead of expressing your anger, sadness, or frustration? Do you have at least one best friend you can count on? People in twelve-step programs have sponsors to call. You can call a friend.

The "I'll Start My Diet Tomorrow" Procrastinator

Have you convinced yourself that you don't have the time to take care of your health? That you are too busy today, but will start tomorrow? Make the time to exercise and cook healthy meals. How much time do you waste a day? Do you watch TV? Do you talk on the telephone with friends and family? Why don't you keep your exercise bike in the middle of the living room, and hop on it whenever you get a call. Or you could dance around the living room while you're watching TV. Stop wasting time!

You may try to make excuses not to exercise. For example, one patient worked part-time from noon to six o'clock in the evening, and she would never get up early to go for a walk. Her excuse was that she liked to watch late night TV. She would sit there and space out in front of the TV and would be too tired to get up and shut it off. So she would watch the TV until two o'clock in the morning when she fell asleep out of sheer exhaustion. Then she couldn't get up in the morning. The answer to her problem is simple: unplug the TV and put it in the closet.

This woman was married to a much younger man. I'm sure she was a knockout in her younger days, but she was looking a bit dowdy. To be honest, with all the extra weight she was carrying, she looked like her husband's mother, not his wife.

The two of them went on a diet together. Well, they were supposed to go on a diet together. He started to eat healthy and exercise. He wasn't doing anything too demanding. He just went out for a brisk walk when he got home from work, or after dinner. He lost a lot of weight and was looking pretty darn handsome.

She, on the other hand, looked the same as she always did. The husband told me that he kept trying to get his wife to go for those walks with him, but she was too busy watching TV. What would you rather do, go for a walk with your handsome, young husband, or watch reruns of *The Love Boat*?

If you have to think twice about the answer to that question, you have a TV addiction and need to do something about it.

The Food Addict

Do you have an eating disorder?

Do you continue to eat even when you're full? (My sister has a really good description for this: she says that her stomach is full, but her mouth is still hungry.)

Do you remain overweight to keep people away from you?

Do you use your weight as an excuse to avoid success?

Do you have deep-seated psychological scars that stem from an unhappy childhood?

Do you eat because you life is controlled by other people, and food is the only thing you can control?

Do you "eat your emotions"?

These are problems that a diet will not cure. Perhaps you need a support group or one-on-one therapy with a psychologist. If you eat because you are depressed, a psychiatrist or even your primary care physician can give you a prescription for an antidepressant, though it may not be enough. You might also need psychotherapy, but an antidepressant is a start.

I'll tell you when I realized I had a problem. I love to cook for people. One morning, there was a spider in my bathroom. Not my favorite of God's creatures, but one of God's creatures nonetheless. Not wanting to kill him, I started talking to the spider. The spider needed to know that there was nothing in the bathroom to eat and that he'd die in there. I asked the spider if he was hungry and began wondering what I had in the refrigerator that a spider might like to eat. At that moment, I realized the depth of my food obsession.

If you know you have a problem but refuse to deal with it, you no longer belong in the "Food Addict" category. Congratulations! You graduated to the "Procrastinator" category.

The Doormat

You know who you are, and you know exactly who is taking advantage of you. Put your foot down. Get some confidence, and stand up for yourself. Banish unhealthy food from the house. You need to sit down and talk to the people in your life. Their psychological issues cause them to sabotage your success. They are afraid they will lose you if you become thin and attractive. Do not let anyone get in your way! Reassure them too. They need to know that you aren't going to leave. If they love you, they will work with you, not against you.

The Caretaker

This is the woman who takes care of everyone but herself. Somehow, "users" seem to find "caretakers." It's all give and no take. This will be hard—but do not answer the phone! Change your phone number. Think about the words to that disco song: Change your locks and make him leave his keys. Everyone will get the message eventually, and so will you. You need to get out of these very unhealthy and psychologically damaging patterns of pain. Users are bottomless pits of need. They will suck you dry. Get out of those relationships; they could kill you. Relationships aren't just about the negatives. Others need to learn they cannot dump on you, but you need to learn a lesson too. You have to draw boundary lines and surround yourself with light, air, energy, and love. Surround yourself with people who wake up in the morning happy to be alive.

Some of you may have taken "caretaker syndrome" to the extreme. Your psychological problems cause you to stay in relationships that are unhealthy, abusive, unfulfilling, or destructive. You think you're taking care of the other person, but all that's happening is that you're being used and abused. Read books like

Codependent No More or *Women Who Love Too Much*. Go to an Al-Anon meeting for codependent family members of alcoholics and, while you're at it, go to Overeaters Anonymous too. Get into therapy. You need to take care of yourself before you can take care of anyone else.

The Self-Defeatist

This is the person who does not believe in herself or the power she has over her own life. There is a beautiful patient who comes to our clinic who is short and morbidly obese. When she started pushing 400 pounds, she got her act together and went into an obesity rehabilitation center for a couple of months. She lost a few pounds there, but really started losing the weight when she got home. She's inching down toward 300 pounds, but now she is claiming, "I cannot get below 300. Every time I get to 300 pounds, I gain all the weight back."

The words you put into the universe will come true. Instead of saying, "I cannot do it," start saying, "I am fabulous. I will lose weight and get below 300 pounds and be even more fabulous." Every morning when you wake up, exclaim, "I am fabulous, life is fabulous, and today is another chance to work toward being healthy."

The Sensitive Soul

A patient once told me that one of her downfalls was eating in restaurants. She and her family ate out frequently. Everyone around her in the restaurant would be eating steaks, cheeseburgers, french fries, and chocolate cake. She was embarrassed to order healthy food because then everyone would know she was on a diet.

I told her about the time I went to the Arnold Classic, a body-building show, with my good friend, Dr. Judy. At the time, I was going through a phase of weight lifting. I wanted to look like one of those models from the pages of a fitness magazine. Needless to say, the phase didn't last long, but it lasted long enough for me to go to the Arnold Classic. Dr. Judy, being the good friend that she is, agreed to let me drag her along. The restaurants, before and after the show, were filled with spectators and participants. Everyone was in really good shape. (You know the type, the muscle heads who shave their chests so that they can show off their sculpted definition.) You could see what everyone was eating: salads, grilled fish, and fruit. They glared in disgust at the few souls eating cheeseburgers. So I told that patient to change her attitude. She needed to be *proud* of her healthy-eating habits. Everyone else in the restaurant was wrong. She was right.

So change your attitude. Be proud! You are a role model for those unhealthy folks who eat cheeseburgers and french fries and then complain about their weight.

The Housewife

Another common excuse is that there is "too much housework" to do. One of my patients liked a clean house. She did laundry and housework in the morning, laundry and housework after work, and more laundry and housework after dinner. She had no time for herself whatsoever.

Twenty years from now, she will still be overweight but will also suffer from hypertension and diabetes. Maybe she will look back and wish she had taken better care of herself. Her house may have been clean and the laundry spick-and-span, but her health suffered. You know, no one ever killed their kids by making them wear a pair of jeans twice in a row. But, you're not doing your children any favors if you feed them junk and don't get them out playing soccer, swimming, running, and generally being vital, healthy, athletic, and full of energy.

What do you want on your tombstone? "Beloved wife, mother, and sister. She kept a clean house"? Or "Beloved wife, mother, and sister. She was fabulous and a great inspiration to us all"?

The Accountant

The accountant believes it's too expensive to diet. Well, it *is* too expensive if you believe all the hype, go out to the supermarket, and buy frozen diet meals. It's too expensive if you buy low-carb breads, diet bars, and liquid meals. It's too expensive to eat out at restaurants and fast-food joints all the time. It's too expensive if you join one of those diet clubs where you have to buy their food.

Dried beans, fruits in season, green leafy vegetables, salad greens, yams, potatoes for baking, winter squash, frozen spinach, fruit, brown rice, whole wheat pasta—these are not expensive foods. For just a few dollars, you can buy a package of dried split peas, carrots, celery, and onions for a delicious soup that would feed a family of four for dinner—twice! You'll need to get creative and spend some time cooking and preparing meals. It will take time and energy. It may even mean less time for watching reruns on Nick at Nite. Heaven forbid! Do whatever it takes because being unhealthy is the most expensive state of being.

So sit and think about where you fit into the above categories. I'm sure that I missed a few. Make your own category, and then find your solution. Aren't you tired of being a housewife, a caretaker, a procrastinator, a doormat, a victim? Aren't you tired of making excuses? Aren't you tired of being tired? I tell my patients that they are their own worst enemy, and all they need to do is get out of their own way. Perhaps everyone needs a source of inspiration.

One of my patients sent me a link to the web site of the Reverend Sue Brockway, an interfaith minister. Her web site has a list of goddesses from cultures throughout history and from around the world. Reverend Brockway believes we can find inspiration from these goddesses. It's not about dancing naked in the forest under a full moon. It's about looking to role models for tips on how to live, love, and be loved. There are goddesses of love, like Venus, who can help you unleash your sensuous side. There are goddesses of war, like the Hindu goddess Durga. Well, war doesn't sound very goddesslike! We are women, after all, and women are supposed to be peaceful and placid. Yet, those of you out there who are codependent can learn a lesson or two from the goddesses of war. You need to draw a line in the sand and protect yourself. Leave it to the

Vikings to combine their goddesses of sex and war into one: Freya. She was a powerhouse. You too need to become aware of your own power.

For those of you with financial issues, there are goddesses of fortune, like the Hindu goddess Lakshmi. Women need to plan for the future. Women need to be empowered. Go for that promotion! You can be a success at work. If you hate your job, go back to school. Change careers. Or if Lakshmi isn't quite your speed, try Isis. This Egyptian mother-goddess brought her husband back from the dead. It's about healing relationships that seem damaged beyond repair. If you decide the relationship isn't worth saving, there is Persephone. She was the woman who was so beautiful that Hades, god of the Underworld, kidnapped her. He carried her down into his realm, where she must spend four months of each year. Without her beauty, the world is cast into cold, dark winter, but when she emerges, springtime blossoms forth. You can liberate yourself from a bad relationship. There is a world of sunshine beyond the cold, dark, and lonely life you're stuck in. You can find the way. Let Nemesis, the Greek goddess of retribution, help you see how you sabotage your relationships and your successes.

There are multiple goddesses throughout history that remind you to love yourself. You cannot take care of anyone unless you take care of yourself. I'm not saying to buy a new Louis Vuitton purse when there is no money in the bank and no food in the refrigerator. Think about your spiritual needs: love, recognition, appreciation, fulfillment, compassion, serenity, inspiration, creativity, and security.

The point is to practice some introspection. Find the beauty and power within yourself. Figure out which goddess you are or aspire to be. Remake yourself. Become a new self. Get out of your own way. Realize that you are a goddess. But even goddesses need to set some goals.

Chapter Four

Goals

Presidents, CEOs, athletes, and most other successful people have specific goals in mind and work every day toward achieving those goals. They wake up every morning and ask, "What will I do today to come closer to my goals?" They have a whole set of goals, both short-term and long-term. They create a game plan and have a timetable laid out for achieving their goals. You can do it too.

First, figure out where you're starting.

> I cannot walk up a flight of stairs without stopping ten times.

> I am 100 pounds overweight.

Second, create your goals based on that starting point, with *benchmarks*. A benchmark is something that is measurable, so that you can rate yourself and track your progress.

> In one month: walk up one flight of stairs without stopping.

> In two months: walk up two flights of stairs without stopping.

> In six months: sign up for kickboxing.

In one year: dance to salsa music at the office holiday party in a tight, red dress.

Third, the real work begins. You need to make a reasonable timetable for your progress in order to achieve your goal. For the sample goal of "walk up one flight of stairs without stopping," you would make a little schedule of all the steps you need to get there:

Week One:

> Day One: Walk around the block once at my own pace.
>
> Day Two: Walk around the block twice at my own pace.
>
> Day Three: Walk around the block four times at my own pace.
>
> By the end of the week: Walk around the block four times as fast as possible.

Week Two:

> Day One: Walk around the block four times, and climb one flight of stairs slowly, stopping as many times as needed.

You get the general picture. Keep going until you reach your goal.

Review your milestones and benchmarks daily, weekly, and monthly. Keep them in the forefront of your mind every day. Write those goals down on Post-it notes and put one on your computer, your desk, the refrigerator, the bathroom mirror, and in your schedule book. If you have a friend who owns a DVD called *The Secret*, you should borrow it. It's about living life in a particular way to achieve your dreams. One of its tips is to draw a picture of the thing that you want and tape the picture to the ceiling. If health and happiness are your goals, choose a photo that best illustrates health and happiness for you. Tape it to the ceiling, so it's the first thing you see when you open your eyes in the morning.

The first thing on your mind when you wake up should be,

"What am I doing today to get healthier?" When you go to sleep at night, you should know that tomorrow is "day two of week two." That's the day you'll be walking around the block four times, and walking up a flight of stairs. It should be the most important thing you do that day. Make it the first thing you do, and not the last. If you put off exercising until the end of the day, you'll never do it. Keep your eye on the light at the end of the tunnel.

Notice that all of the goals we talked about have something to do with activity. Don't worry about your weight. Worry about your health. Don't set weight goals; set activity goals.

So make your short-term and long-term goals:

I am now	
In 4 weeks, I will be	
In 8 weeks, I will be	
In 12 weeks, I will be	
In 1 year, I will be	
In 5 years, I will be	
In 20 years, I will be	

Set Realistic Goals

You cannot make a goal of losing 20 pounds in a month! No one should go on a crash diet. If weight loss is your goal, a good rule of thumb is to lose 1 percent of your body weight per week. For a 250-pound woman, that would be a goal of 2 ½ pounds per week, max. You don't need such an ambitious goal. Even 1 pound a week or a pound every other week would be 25 to 50 pounds in a year. That's not such a bad goal! We're making lifestyle changes; we're not going on crash diets here. Focus on your health, not on your weight.

Remember, your weight is your weight for how much you exercise and how much you eat right now. Let me explain. There are patients who have been coming to the clinic for years. For some patients, their weight has been steady as a rock for years. A pound up or down here and there, but, overall, the same. This is how much they weigh for how much they eat and exercise. Their weight reflects their lifestyle, the food they eat, how much they exercise, and the genes they inherited from their parents. This is called the "set-point weight."

For other patients, when I review their charts, we see a steady and constant weight gain through the years. One woman has been coming to the clinic for years. She has gained 6 pounds a year for the past ten years. She hasn't even hit her set-point weight yet! This reflects her lifestyle: she eats more than she burns off every day. She weighed 160 pounds ten years ago when she was twenty-one years old. Now she weighs 220 pounds at thirty-one. She was horrified when we did the math. In ten years, when she turns forty-one years old, she is going to weigh 280 pounds. Ten years after that, when she turns fifty-one years old, she will weigh 340 pounds. She will continue to gain weight at the rate of 6 pounds per year unless she makes some serious changes to her lifestyle. People gravitate to a weight that reflects how much they eat and how much they exercise.

A better example is my cousin's husband, Stan. He grew up on a dairy farm. Dairy farmers work hard, really hard. They milk the cows twice a day, 365 days a year. Whether it's hot or cold, raining or snowing, the cows need to be milked. The farmers move the cows from pasture to pasture during the spring and summer, and they grow grass to make hay to feed the animals during the winter. Every night at dinner, the guys on the farm ate a loaf of bread, each! When Stan went away to college, he wasn't milking the cows anymore, and he wasn't baling hay. He was sitting around studying, and eating a loaf of bread every night with dinner. He came back for Christmas vacation that first year and went to go visit his future wife, my cousin Gina. When she opened the door, she was shocked and blurted out, "What happened to you?" She says that it looked as if someone had pumped him up with air, like a balloon. He hadn't changed his eating habits at all. He was eating the exact same amount of food he had always eaten, but he wasn't getting any exercise. But, that was a long time ago, and he is in great shape now.

Let me emphasize it again: people gravitate to a weight that reflects how much they eat and how much they exercise. It just goes to show you that you cannot go back to your old exercise and eating habits. You need to make lifestyle changes that are permanent; otherwise, you will gravitate back to your old weight and your old body. Since the goal is fitness and health, put a plan into action that includes physical activity every day as well as time to prepare healthy meals.

You can set ambitious goals, but be prepared to work at them.

Make New Friends

If you look at your five closest friends and relatives, you can see a reflection of yourself: how much you earn, your religious affiliation, your political party, and how much you weigh. If the five people closest to you are couch potatoes, you will be too. If, instead, those five people are high energy and goal oriented, you might get inspired. Make some new friends that are into health and fitness. It will rub off on you.

Track Your Progress

Keep a log. Get a little notebook, and make it your diary. Put your short-term and long-term goals on the front page. Track your daily exercise and food intake. Write down your feelings and your frustrations.

There are a few reasons to do this. First of all, it will help you keep track of your calories. Counting calories is not for everyone. As a matter of fact, it's a pain in the neck. But if you are obese, I strongly recommend counting calories. You won't need to do it forever. Do it for a few weeks. You need to learn how many calories are in the foods you eat, and you need to learn portion sizes. If you continue to eat more than you can burn off, you'll be like our friend who has been gaining 6 pounds a year for the past ten years. Sometimes, writing down all the food you eat in a day can help you see where you can make small changes. Small changes add up over time.

Another reason for the log is to plan your day ahead of time. You need to be prepared to have breakfast, lunch, dinner, and a snack or two throughout the day. While you don't need to know you will be eating precisely one ounce of walnuts and an orange at exactly three o'clock tomorrow, you do need to plan your day in advance so you can have a snack packed in your bag.

If you have a pedometer, track your steps in the log. Aim for ten thousand steps every day. There are some heavy patients who eat very little; I would starve on what they eat. The difference is they get no exercise whatsoever. Their food log tells us they need to get out and get moving.

The most important reason to keep the log is the satisfaction and inspiration it will give you as you track your progress. If you're obese or overweight, you are actually starting out ahead. It means you love food. You love to eat. You love life. This is a good thing. Channel that energy and love into planning your meals and preparing healthy foods for you and your family. Make health and fitness the center of your universe. Turn your obsession with food from a negative into a positive trait.

Chapter Five

Put Your Body on a Schedule

Here is what one patient wrote in her food log for two days:

Day One

        11:30 a.m. Sausage, garlic bread

        1:00 p.m. Pig's feet, potato salad, dumplings

        8:00 p.m. Stewed chicken, rice and beans

Day Two

        9:30 a.m. Cheese, eggs, sausage, bread, butter

        4:10 p.m. Black beans, rice, fried pork chops, tripe soup

        9:00 p.m. Avocado salad with oil and vinegar

What is wrong with this picture? Yes, yes. There aren't many vegetables. What else?

She's not on any schedule! You can almost see her sitting in her living room watching TV until a lightbulb goes off in her head…"I'm hungry!" She then trots over to the kitchen, opens the refrigerator door, and stares at its contents, trying to figure out what to eat. She had not planned to get hungry. She had not planned to have dinner ready.

I see this over and over again in my practice—disorganized lifestyles and haphazard eating patterns. There isn't any planning for meals or meal times; so many people just grab whatever is quick and easy. Sometimes they wait so long to eat that they are ravenous by the time they sit down for dinner. Using my patient above as an example, she must have been really hungry by the time she ate lunch on Day Two because there were almost seven hours between breakfast and lunch.

On this program, you'll be eating *four*, *five*, or even *six* times a day: three meals and a snack or two.

Eating every few hours is important. Try to stick to a normal schedule of meal times. Your body will become accustomed to the routine of normal-sized meals at normal times. The point is to never get overly hungry. When you wait to eat until you're starving, you overeat.

Let me give you a few examples. I once practiced in Fredericksburg, Virginia, and many of my patients worked in Washington, DC—a sixty-mile commute each way. One mom would drop her kids off at school in the morning and then commute to DC, so she could be at work by nine o'clock. She had decided, after eating too much for dinner one night, to start her diet once again. She was serious this time, so breakfast was an apple or a packet of instant oatmeal. Lunch was a low-fat turkey sandwich or one of those frozen diet meals. At five o'clock in the afternoon, she would get into her car to head home. Her stomach was grumbling. She was hungry. By the time she would get home at six thirty, she was *really* hungry. She would start preparing dinner for her family, but she was ravenous. She couldn't control her hunger and would eat way too much of anything she could grab. No wonder! She starved herself throughout the day. One apple and a low-fat turkey sandwich would not get me past ten o'clock in the morning, let alone seven o'clock in the evening.

Missed meals, not eating enough food (like an apple for breakfast), or long stretches of time between meals are not allowed. Starving is not allowed. It's amazing how many people eat lunch at noon and expect to wait until seven or eight in the evening to eat dinner. They're starving by that time—then eat too much, too quickly.

In a later chapter, we will talk about counting calories. As I said before, it's not for everybody; some people can do it, and some people cannot. One of the benefits of counting calories is that it helps you plan and prepare for your day. If that mom had looked at the calories on the frozen meal, she would have realized it was only 300 calories, and the apple she had for breakfast was 100 calories. An average woman might need around 1,600 calories a day, more if she is overweight, less if she is petite. More if she exercises (the elite bicyclists who compete in the Tour de France probably eat 16,000 calories a day during the race!), less if she is a couch potato.

Use 1,600 calories per day as a road map to plan your meals. Spread out the calories over time—*100 calories for every hour that you're awake.* Eating 400 calories each for breakfast, lunch, and dinner, plus two 200-calorie snacks, is a good approach. Alternatively, you could do four 400-calorie meals. So earlier, when I wrote that you should eat roughly five times a day, I did not mean five full-sized meals. These really need to be three normal-sized meals and two small snacks. It's important to spread out your calories through the day. It doesn't matter how you decide to do it, as long as it's reasonable and the food is not all clumped into one big meal.

Depending on your life and your schedule, you could start with one of these variations:

For a teacher working from eight in the morning to three in the afternoon,

Breakfast: 7:00 a.m.
Lunch: 11:30 a.m.
Snack: 3:30 p.m.
Dinner: 7:00 p.m.

For someone working twelve-hour shifts from eight in the morning to eight in the evening,

Breakfast: 7:00 a.m.
Lunch: Noon
Large Snack: 4:00 p.m.
Light Dinner: 8:00 p.m.

For a nine-to-five worker with a long commute, like our friend in Virginia,

Breakfast: 7:00 a.m.
Small snack: 10:00 a.m.
Lunch: Noon
Snack: 4:00 p.m.
Dinner: 7:00 p.m.

The purpose of spreading out your meals is so you *don't go hungry!* Eat when you are hungry. Don't try to starve yourself; it always backfires in the long run. The urge to eat is no different from the urge to go to the bathroom. You have no control over basic bodily urges. You must eat when you're hungry; otherwise, you will spin out of control and grab anything to eat. Isn't it better to eat healthy food at the first pangs of hunger than to gorge yourself when you become wild from starvation?

Do you know someone who went on a liquid diet and lost a tremendous amount of weight? Were they happy? I doubt it, because it's hard to be happy when you're hungry. Did they gain all the weight back? I bet they did, plus some.

When you start a strict diet, you put yourself into starvation mode, and a few things happen. As starvation mode kicks in, the body starts burning muscle for energy. If you fall into a pattern of eating too little for breakfast and lunch and then overeating at dinner, over time you slowly alter the fat-to-lean proportion of your body. Your weight may remain the same, but your body fat percentage continually increases and your muscle mass decreases.

Personal trainers and nutritionists have coined a term: skinny-fat. People who are skinny-fat may be thin, but they have no muscle tone and a high percentage of body fat. Our mom in Virginia had only eaten 400 calories over the first twelve hours of the day. If she then ate 1,200 calories for dinner, she would have only eaten 1,600 calories that day. That's a very reasonable number of calories for a day. But the body cannot burn 1,200 calories of food all at once, so the excess is stored as fat. She is changing her ratio of muscle to fat over time: losing muscle and gaining fat, a little bit every day. Over time, the changes accumulate, and she becomes skinny-fat. It's far healthier to spread your calories throughout the day. The purpose of eating healthy is to look good and feel good. What's the use of dieting if you're turning yourself into flab?

Starving yourself also slows down how fast you burn calories. The body becomes more and more efficient at using calories. You have to eat less and less in order to maintain the same body weight. For instance, a famous supermodel had a baby a few years ago. Right after she gave birth, she put herself on a 600-calorie-a-day diet, so she could get back to her pre-pregnancy weight in a few weeks. What a bad idea! Some patients tell me that when they want to lose weight, they eat only one meal a day. That's an even worse idea!

So start planning. Be on a schedule. Don't starve for two hours in your car or on the subway and then pig out at dinner. You need to have a schedule of breakfast, lunch, dinner, and a snack or two.

You need to start organizing your life, and your eating habits.

Chapter Six

Get Moving! The Road to Obesity Starts at Your TV

There is some fascinating new research looking at the inner workings of the brains of people who suffer from obesity. If you just look at an MRI or a CT scan of the brains of thin and obese people, their brains would look alike. MRIs and CTs show the shape and size of the brain. They would show a stroke or a tumor, but they would not tell us anything about brain *activity*. To look at activity in the brain, there are high-tech machines called PET (Positron Emission Tomography) scanners. Different parts of the brain have different functions. If you're adding up the grocery bill, one area of the brain lights up. If you're listening to music, a different area lights up. Scientists can look at which areas of the brain light up when you eat or exercise, or even just think about eating or exercising.

One area of the brain, the right prefrontal cortex, is located in the front of the brain, on the right side. This area is less active in the brains of people who are obese and sedentary. For people who are physically active, their right prefrontal cortex is more active. In athletes, this area lights up like a Christmas tree on PET scans. So, scientists think that this area of the brain is involved in motivating people to move. If you don't like to exercise, your right prefrontal cortex may be telling you to sit around and watch TV. Well, maybe your right prefrontal cortex isn't exactly telling you to watch TV, but it isn't telling you to go out for a walk either.

The good news is that when you start becoming more physically active, the right prefrontal cortex grows and starts to light up on the PET scan. This is called the *plasticity* of the brain, which means that it can change. If your brain can change, so can you. Let's twist that old saying around from, "the less you do, the less you want to do" to a new one: "The more you do, the more you want to do."

Exercise is the most important lifestyle change you can make, even more important than dieting. Let's look at a couple of examples to illustrate this, starting with ducks and ending with sumo wrestlers. When ducks, geese, or any migrating birds prepare for the long trip south before the winter, they start packing on the pounds in the late summer and early autumn. They scarf down as many fruits and nuts as they can. The birds need to store plenty of fat; they will need it to get them through the long trip. Migrating birds fly hundreds of miles every day, and that requires a lot of energy. (And you complain about walking to the post office?)

All those extra calories from fruits and nuts are stored as fat in the liver and inside the abdominal cavity. The fat inside the abdominal cavity is also called visceral fat. This is *fast fat*. Visceral fat is very metabolically active. The body can mobilize visceral fat quickly to use as energy on those long journeys. People store fat in the exact same way, in the liver and the abdominal cavity, getting ready for the long winter migration. But we aren't going anywhere—except maybe the hospital. Belly fat, stored inside the abdominal cavity, is associated with diabetes. It's part of the process leading not only to diabetes but also to hypertension, high cholesterol, heart disease, and strokes.

Just like the migrating birds, sumo wrestlers are great examples of the importance of exercise as well. These 400-pound men are at high risk for diabetes, but not until after they retire from wrestling. If you do an MRI or CT scan of their bellies while they are still actively wrestling, they have no belly fat. (Remember, belly fat is associated with diabetes.) All of their fat while they are still active is in their subcutaneous (i.e., under the skin) tissue.[1] The training for sumo wrestlers is very vigorous. They spend hours every day doing their exercise regimens. When they retire, they stop doing all that activity. One year after retirement, if you do another CT, it will show that all of the fat has shifted from under the skin into the belly. This is when the wrestlers start getting diabetes—when they stop exercising! And so, exercise may be even *more* important than what or how much you eat.

You don't need to start wrestling. Just start by walking, even for a few minutes, or a few blocks. Do it with your family, a neighbor, a friend…anyone. People who start an exercise program with a partner are ten times more likely to stick to it over the long haul. Use that time to build relationships. Walk every day with your husband, wife, life partner, children, sisters, brothers, or friends.

A few years ago, a friend and I went on a group expedition to remote islands in Polynesia. We went from island to island on a large sailboat. When we reached an island, we would transfer onto little motorboats, ride through the reef, land on the beach, and hike through the island. One hike was up the side of a (hopefully) extinct volcano. The walk was hard and treacherous. Even though I was in excellent shape at the time, this hike up the side of the mountain was *hard*. Every time I looked down to plan my next step up, sweat would drip from my forehead. When we reached the top, my friend plopped down on a rock, and I plopped down next to her. We were sweaty, dirty, and out of breath, but we were proud of ourselves. Next to arrive at the top was a tall, blond Swedish woman. Not a drop of sweat was on her forehead, and her

---

1. A. D. Karelis and others, "Metabolic and Body Composition Factors in Subgroups of Obesity: What Do We Know?" *Clinical Endocrinology and Metabolism* 89, no. 6 (2004): 2569–2575.

white tennis skirt was still spotless. Close behind the Viking lady was a couple: he was eighty-two, and she was eighty-three. They were talking and laughing. I couldn't believe it! They must have been Olympic athletes in their youth, or marathon runners, or astronauts!

Not even close. The next day, after I had recuperated, we sat together and had a wonderful conversation. He was a retired diplomat, and she was a homemaker. They had one secret: they walked together one hour a day, every day, except during thunderstorms and blizzards. Not a leisurely, window-shopping-pace stroll, but a good hearty walk. They got their hearts pumping and blood flowing *just one hour a day*—and that walk improved the quality of their entire life. That one hour, when they walked and talked together every day and gave each other full attention, also helped them sustain a happy marriage for sixty years.

In Nordic countries, like Sweden and Finland, where it's winter six months of the year, and in Canada, where strawberry season is in August, you would think that everyone stays indoors when it's cold. You would think people gain weight during the winter, but it's just the opposite. In those countries, even during the winter, people get out and move. People skate, ski, snowshoe, or just walk. No one belongs to a gym. Everyone suits up in warm clothes and goes outside to play or work. There are no excuses.

Here is another story, closer to home. One of my former patients is young; she is in her thirties. She had been quite obese but had not been to the clinic in over a year. One day, we passed each other on the street. She was wearing a gray-blue uniform from the postal service, and she was unrecognizable, a shadow of her former self. She was fifty pounds lighter thanks to the walking she did all day, five days a week.

Getting a job as a mail carrier may not be an option for you, but you can still get out there and walk! If a couple in their eighties can do it, and millions of people who live in freezing cold climates can do it, so can you. Just drop the excuses:

"It's too hot."

"It's too cold."

"There are no sidewalks where I live."

"It's raining."

"I'm too fat to leave the house."

"I'll miss reruns of *The Jeffersons*."

You don't want to leave the house? Okay, but find an activity you can do in your house. You can almost always find an exercise class on cable TV, if you do some channel surfing. One of my patients told me there are "on-demand" exercise classes on cable TV. You can watch on-demand exercise classes just like on-demand movies. She can choose anything from hip-hop to belly dancing! Do a class every day. When you can't find free on-demand exercise classes on TV, drag your old exercise bike out from under that pile of dirty laundry in the far corner of your bedroom. Don't have a bike? Borrow a friend's. Everybody knows someone with an old exercise bike, and they will be happy to get rid of it. Put that old bike in the middle of the living room and bike while you watch TV. Hop on the bike when you get a phone call.

Still can't get a bike? Don't like to bike? Then step in place while you're watching TV. Put on some music, and dance around the apartment. Rent or buy some exercise videotapes. Depending on your age, you could rock to the oldies with Richard Simmons, or dance with Jane Fonda, or kick some Tae Bo butt. If aerobics or kickboxing is not your speed, try belly dancing. Belly dancing is very empowering for women of substance. It helps you get in touch with your inner goddess.

Don't want to exercise at home? Go out dancing with some friends. Don't want to go out to dance but still love to boogie? You could organize a weekly dance party with friends and rotate apartments.

What about joining a gym? Wait to join. First of all, some gyms are unscrupulous and will try to rip you off. Before you join, research the gym on the Better Business Bureau web site. Many gyms will lock you into a three-year contract and then sue you if you fall behind on payments. Second, do not join unless you have a workout partner who will go with you; otherwise, you'll never get out of the house and off to the gym. Lastly, you don't need to spend money on a gym membership. You can complete a pretty good workout without fancy machines. Use the money you save by not joining a gym on healthy fruits and vegetables!

Exercise may be easier said than done. Some of my patients cannot walk more than a block or two. They are so out of shape that even walking a block makes them short of breath. Their knees and hips have severe arthritis from years of carrying around an extra 100 to 200 pounds. Even to them, I say, keep moving. If you cannot walk, put on some music. Sit and move along with the beat as best you can. You'll eventually get there.

There is no excuse for not exercising.

Do *something*, anything. Just keep moving!

Chapter Seven

Exercise: Aerobic and Resistance

W
e already discussed your set-point weight. This is how much you weigh for how much you eat and how much you exercise. *Basal metabolic rate* is another term you'll hear when you talk about weight. Basal metabolic rate, or BMR, is the number of calories you burn while completely at rest. It's how much you need to eat to maintain your current weight if you do nothing except sit around and breathe. So, what does basal metabolic rate have to do with losing weight? What does it mean to you if you're trying to lose a pound a week?

There are 3,500 calories stored in a pound of fat. In order to lose a pound of fat, you would need to eat 3,500 less calories. You could do that by not eating anything for two days. Not a good idea. More realistically, by eating 500 calories less a day, you would lose a pound in one week (500 x 7 = 3,500). So, stop drinking that soda and you'll be as thin as a supermodel in no time! Well, maybe not as thin, but you'll still be healthier than you are now.

When you diet, you cut down the number of calories you eat every day, and your BMR slows down. As a matter of fact, if you lose 10 percent of your body weight, your BMR actually slows down by 18 to 22 percent. If you weigh 250 pounds and slim down to 225, you lost 10 percent of your body weight. So instead of your old calorie intake of, let's say, 2,000 calories per day, it would make sense that you should be eating 10 percent less, or 1,800 calories per day, to maintain your new body. Well, it doesn't work like that. Your BMR has slowed down, so you need to eat closer to 1,600 calories every day to maintain the new weight. You need to reduce your calories by close to 20 percent to maintain your new 10 percent thinner body. Now why would our bodies try to sabotage our diet plan? Don't our bodies know we are trying to lose weight? Why doesn't that stupid BMR go up when we diet? We want to eat more and weigh less.

Well, that slowdown in BMR happens for a very good reason. It's part of our survival mechanism. It's hardwired into our genes. When you diet by cutting down on calories, the body goes into survival mode. It reacts the same way it did tens of thousands, hundreds of thousands, or millions of years ago when food was scarce, like during famines, droughts, and winters. When you decrease the amount of food you eat every day, your body thinks another winter is coming. Your body slows down the amount of food it needs so that you can survive the long winter.

Remember that back in the old days, life was either a feast or a famine. The men went out hunting, and one of three things happened:

1. They got lost. (Even back then, do you think men ever asked for directions?)

2. They came back with no food.

3. They came back with a lot of food.

You never knew when the men were going to come back empty-handed or with a woolly mammoth. When you diet today, your body thinks a famine is coming; it thinks another winter is just around the corner, with no food for months at a time. Your BMR slows down to protect you from starvation.

This protective mechanism has helped humans survive through thousands of long frozen winters. But today, there aren't any famines in America anymore. We can eat warm cherry pie in the middle of the winter or ice cream in the middle of the summer. When it rains, we can telephone Chinese takeout, so we don't need to walk any further than the front door for dinner. We can pull out a frozen dinner and stick it in the microwave in case we become hungry in the middle of the night. Every day is a feast. A slower BMR means something different for us.

After losing weight by going on a diet, you can never go back to your old eating habits. For example, let's say you weigh 250 pounds. You probably eat 2,500 or even 3,000 calories a day to maintain that weight. Then, you go on a diet and slim down to 225 pounds. You may have done that by eating 250 calories less every day for six months (twenty-five weeks), or by eating 500 calories less every day for three months (twelve and a half weeks). Now you weigh 225. Congratulations! But if you go back to eating 2,500 or 3,000 calories every day (same old food, same old quantity), what do you think is going to happen? That's right, you'll gain back 25 pounds for two reasons:

1. A 225-pound body needs fewer calories to maintain a weight of 225 than it did to maintain a weight of 250 pounds.

2. Your BMR has slowed down. Your body has become a lean, mean, fuel-efficient machine. When you trade in your Hummer for a Honda, you need less gasoline.

You might even gain back more than the 25 pounds you lost because your BMR slowed down. This is the *yo-yo syndrome*. Diet, lose weight, gain back more, diet, lose weight, and gain back more, etc. This is why diets don't work. You need permanent changes to the foods you eat; they need to be both healthy and satisfying. You need to find healthy foods you enjoy, healthy foods you don't mind eating for the rest of your life!

Can you do anything about your BMR? Can you increase it with exercise? The myth is that if you exercise, your BMR increases. This myth also says that you burn calories for a full twenty-four hours after you exercise, meaning you could do a workout on Monday, lay around on the couch all day on Tuesday, and still burn extra calories. Well, like everything else about the human body, it just isn't that simple. Exercise may or may not increase your BMR. It depends on how hard you exercise and for how long. Exercise physiologists have found that to increase your BMR an extra twenty-four hours after an exercise, you need to exercise *hard* for at least fifty minutes. If you are out of shape, don't try this at home. You'll give yourself a heart attack. The only people who can really do this are athletes, runners, or people who do an intense aerobic exercise on a regular basis.

You can do it too, but it will take time to get there. In the meanwhile, as you're working up to exercising at greater and greater intensities, you will still lose weight. The calories you burn might only be the calories that you burn during the time you exercise. You might not burn *extra* calories for another twenty-four hours after you stop, but that's okay.

On the other hand, if you are a diabetic and do a one-hour session of resistance exercise, your muscles will absorb sugar from the bloodstream more efficiently for the next twenty-four hours. That's right. Your muscles would be less insulin-resistant for a whole day. Your blood sugar would be under better control. If you have diabetes, you should consider exercise every single day as part of your plan to control your blood sugar.

So get out there. You can walk, dance, chase the kids—anything that strikes your fancy. Just keep moving! That's why it's so important to find an exercise that you enjoy. If going to the gym and walking on the treadmill bores you to tears, you will not be able to do it for the rest of your life. Find something you like to do, and find someone to do it with. Near my house, there is a small field. Every day after work, there are people playing ball:

handball, baseball, football, soccer, or volleyball. One day, there was a whole family playing soccer together. Three generations of the family, men and women, were playing, including the toddlers. The toddlers never really kicked the ball. They were just running back and forth, chasing after the adults, the ball, and each other. The whole family got a good workout, and had a lot of fun at the same time.

Aerobic Exercise

Aerobic exercise is any exercise that increases your heart rate, like running, jogging, brisk walking, kickboxing, rowing, biking, swimming, tennis, jumping rope, step aerobics, jumping jacks, or playing soccer with your family. If you're *moving* and *sweating*, you're doing an aerobic exercise. This is how you are going to mobilize the abdominal fat.

If you pay attention to the science news, you'll know about the recommendations for aerobic exercise, which keep changing: twenty minutes three times a week versus ten minutes every day versus one hour a day. That's all well and good, but so confusing. What the scientists are talking about is the *minimum* exercise required to maintain a *minimum* level of fitness. We don't want a minimum level of fitness. We want to burn fat and be healthy. Walking ten minutes every day won't do much to help you reach your goals.

So how much do we need to exercise in order to lose weight? We could be scientific about it. When scientists talk about heart rates, they will tell you to exercise at a particular percentage of your maximum heart rate. Your maximum heart rate is the fastest your heart can beat. It varies by age. The formula is 220 - your age = maximum heart rate. If you're fifty years old, your maximum heart rate is 170 beats per minute (220 - 50 = 170). The scientific recommendation for aerobic exercise is to increase your heart rate to between 60 and 90 percent of the maximum. For a fifty year old, that would be between 102 and 153 beats per minute. Check the following chart to find out what your target heart rate is.

Age	60%	70%	80%
20	120	140	160
25	117	136	156
30	114	133	152
35	111	130	148
40	108	126	144
45	105	123	140
50	102	119	136
55	99	116	132

Fat burning occurs better at the lower end of your *target* heart rate, at 60 to 70 percent of your maximum heart rate. You burn a greater *percentage* of fat if you walk four miles in one hour at a heart rate of 108 than if you run those four miles in thirty minutes at a heart rate of 153. Don't try to get your heart rate up to 90, 80, or even 70 percent if you are really out of shape. You will give yourself a heart attack.

You can also burn a greater percentage of fat if you exercise in the morning before breakfast. This is when you have the lowest amount of glycogen stored in your muscles and are more likely to burn fat. Glycogen is the body's short-term fuel and is stored in the liver and the muscles. It's made up of sugars with simple single bonds between each sugar. You want to exercise when you have the lowest amounts of glycogen so that the body can burn fat instead of glycogen. The theory is that it takes at least twenty minutes of exercise before one starts to burn fat.

Hence, exercise for *at least* twenty minutes, ideally in the morning when your glycogen stores are the lowest. Notice the very subtle difference between how you burn fat at different heart rates. Exercise at the lower end of your target heart rate burns a greater *percentage* of fat, not more *overall* calories. If a runner runs four miles, and a walker walks four miles, the runner burns more calories than the walker. The people who really care about this are bodybuilders, who need to maintain their muscle mass. Their aerobic exercise is done at a lower heart rate but for a longer period of time. This should not give you carte blanche to exercise below your capability. The bodybuilders will walk on a treadmill for an hour, but they do it at an 11 percent incline. That's very hard work. So, exert yourself. If you do want to try to burn fat by exercising at lower heart rates, remember that you need to exercise for a longer period of time.

Putting it all together, get out and walk, ideally in the morning before breakfast. Exercise aerobically for a minimum of twenty minutes. With a five-minute warm-up at the front end and a five-minute cooldown at the back end, you'll be out there for thirty minutes.

You may have heard of the importance of stretching before exercise. There are proper techniques to stretch. Some people actually hurt themselves stretching by not using proper techniques. If you want to stretch, there is plenty of information, either in books or on the Internet. Stretching is not necessary if all you're doing is walking. You can worry about stretching later, after you become more fit and want to get serious about exercise.

Now, if you really want to burn fat, and you have the time to spend, power walk twice a day. Exercise at 60 percent of your maximum heart rate for sixty minutes: once in the morning before you eat breakfast and again one hour sometime between dinner and bedtime. Watch that fat melt away.

Some people worry about walking after dinner, but *waiting ninety minutes after a meal to work out is a myth*. The only reason to wait is to avoid a stomachache if you are going on a five-mile run. If you're only going out for an after-dinner stroll, there is no need to wait ninety minutes. As a matter of fact, an after-dinner stroll is not such a bad idea. It will get you out of the house, away from the temptation to raid the refrigerator, and away from the TV. It will also act as a reality check. If you cannot walk after dinner, it means that you ate too much.

If you are new to exercise and are very out of shape, you may only get out there for five minutes the first day. Twenty years ago during medical school and my residency, I never went to the gym. All my time was spent working in the hospital, studying, or all too rarely, sleeping. The day after the Internal Medicine Board exam, my life was my own again. The first thing I did that day was sign up at the neighborhood gym. After five minutes on an exercise bike, it was time to go home and take a nap. The next day, the same thing happened: gym time, nap. It only took a couple of months to work up to step aerobics classes. So just be persistent. Keep it up, and don't be discouraged. Don't feel bad if you need a nap after exercising, although you might not to want to exercise before going to work. Your boss will not be happy if you're sleeping at your desk. When you get into better physical condition, you won't need to nap anymore.

Start by walking, with the ultimate goal being at least twenty minutes of aerobic exercise every day. Remember, aerobic exercise is anything that increases your heart rate. The heart is a muscle. When it beats faster, it becomes stronger and more efficient at pumping blood to the body.

So to review, increase your heart rate to between 60 and 90 percent of your maximum heart rate. Keep your heart rate there for at least twenty minutes. If you're really out of shape, and your only exercise is chewing, don't even think about heart rate until you are in better physical condition.

Use the heart rate chart to figure out where your target heart rate is. Or have a friend or your physician teach you how to take your pulse. Adjust your level of exertion to keep your pulse in your target. If you can afford to purchase a wrist heart monitor, great, but save time and money. You don't need to stop every five minutes to check your pulse. You don't need a heart rate monitor. You *know* if you are working hard enough. You *know* whether or not you are sweating. You *know* if you are cheating. Just stop making excuses, and do it. If you want to spend a few dollars, get a pedometer instead of a heart rate monitor. Aim for ten thousand steps a day. Take it over the top: aim for twenty thousand steps a day, and throw a big party when you get there.

Resistance Exercise

The definition of resistance exercise is movement of muscle against a weight. It does not involve pumping blood through your heart, or even getting your heart rate up. It involves using your muscles to lift or move a load. The classic example of resistance exercise is weight lifting, either with free weights or the machines at the gym. Everybody always asks about lifting weights. A few women want to start right away, but most don't want to because they feel that it will make them bulky. Don't worry about bulk. It takes years of extreme dedication and hard work to develop that much muscle. Plus, would you mind looking like Serena or Venus Williams? I wouldn't mind one bit.

So what about resistance exercise? You *want* to build muscle. It used to be believed that by building muscle, you would burn more calories, even at rest. Like the Energizer Bunny, those muscles would keep burning calories 24-7, even after you went to sleep, because your BMR would be increased. Well, research has never proven this, but we all still believe it, though it may not be true. Even if it doesn't help you burn calories while you're sleeping, I'm a big believer in weight lifting. It strengthens bones, ligaments, and tendons; increases strength; and builds muscle as well. If you are a diabetic or prediabetic, resistance exercise helps the muscles pull sugar out of the blood stream for a full twenty-four hours after the exercise.

If your exercise time is limited, just do the aerobic exercise and worry about the weight lifting later. You can start after you have lost weight and want better body definition. If you're ready to start now, concentrate on the body part that is *smaller* than the rest of your body. If you are bottom-heavy, concentrate on building your chest and shoulders. You will look better and more proportional in the long run.

There are a thousand theories on how to lift weights, too many for this short introduction. But there are a few rules.

Watch your form. Do not lift weights sloppily because that's how people injure joints. The purpose is not to throw the weights around. The purpose is to build a strong and healthy body. Lift slowly and carefully. There is a retired professional bodybuilder named Bob Paris. When he lifts, he makes it look like ballet. That's the point. Lift slowly and carefully with perfect form. You're less likely to injure yourself, and you get the maximum benefit from the least amount of weight. Go buy a weight-lifting magazine. Even if you never want to look as muscle-bound as those men and women, there are always articles about the proper way to lift and proper nutrition. Go to the local bookstore or library, and look through the weight-lifting books. There are some good ones out there now. Better yet, every person I know has a son, nephew, boyfriend, cousin, or friend who is interested in bodybuilding. One of them would be thrilled to drag you to the gym twice week and put you through your paces. Don't fight with your newfound coach. Don't argue when he or she tells you to do bicep curls with a 10-pound weight. Just let your coach take over and boss you around in the gym. Do you think that Serena is arguing with her coach, "I don't feel like hitting the ball today. My racket is too heavy. The ball is too small, and it's too hot"? I don't think so!

Never try to lift a weight heavier than your ability. I know you don't want to look silly in the gym, lifting little 5-pound weights while everyone else is bench-pressing 200 pounds. Don't worry about everyone else. If you hurt yourself, it will put your weight-loss regimen back three months. But you still need to lift a weight that's going to make a difference. Doing bicep curls with 2-pound weights is not going to build muscle. Use enough weight so the muscles are stressed. That's how they strengthen and grow. If you can lift the weight ten times easily, it's too light. You should lift a weight that gets really heavy by the tenth repetition. Do three sets of ten repetitions of each exercise.

Sleep Eight Hours a Night

What is sleep doing in the exercise chapter? If you're exercising at the appropriate level of intensity, you will need eight hours of sleep every night. Your muscles need time to repair. You may even need more than eight hours of sleep on some days. Adequate sleep will help your memory too. It's a sad state of affairs we are in. We are all so busy with work, housework, and the kids that sleep has become a luxury. Sleep is a necessity, the same as air, food, and water. Spoil yourself. Sleep eight hours a night.

As an added incentive to get to bed, did you know that *people who are sleep deprived are more likely to be overweight!* Several studies have shown an association between too little sleep and obesity![1] Yes, people who don't get enough sleep tend to be overweight, or even obese. There are hormones in the body whose purpose is to control hunger. When you don't get enough sleep, levels of those hormones change. The sensation of feeling hungry isn't just because your stomach is empty. Hormones secreted by the stomach, small intestine, and fat cells are all working together to send a message to your brain that it's time to eat.

This is a brand new area of research for scientists. Half of those hunger hormones weren't even known twenty years ago. They hadn't been discovered yet. What scientists have found is that if you don't get enough sleep, levels of a hormone called *ghrelin*, which stimulates hunger, goes up. Way up! If that weren't enough to make you hungry, levels of *leptin*, a hormone that helps you feel satisfied, goes down. All you have to do to help move those hormone levels into the right direction is sleep. *Sleep your way to a better body!* There is no excuse for watching stupid TV shows late into the night when you should be sleeping.

Water

Bring water with you if you are going on a long power walk on a hot day. Stay away from all those sports drinks if you're trying to

---

1. N. D. Kohatsu and others, "Sleep Duration and Body Mass Index in a Rural Population," *Archives of Internal Medicine* 166 (2006): 1701–1705.

lose weight; they are high in calories. The purpose of those sports drinks is to replace the electrolytes, like potassium and sodium, that people lose when they sweat a lot during vigorous exercise. Marathon runners, especially if they are running on a hot day, can lose so much sodium in their sweat that the level of sodium in their blood goes down also. When that happens, they become nauseated and light-headed. It's hard to finish running a twenty-six-mile race when you don't feel good!

If you're just starting out exercising, you probably don't have to worry about sodium levels in your bloodstream. You're not going to be exercising hard enough to lose sodium. Just get out there and walk. Worry about electrolytes when you start training for the marathon.

If you hate walking, and you hate exercising, and you hate sweating, well, I don't know what to tell you. You'll need to just accept yourself the way you are.

Chapter Eight

GM Is Not Just a Car Company (Genetically Modified Foods and Trans Fats)

ats and oils in your diet are essential for good health.[1] The body needs *lipids*, another term for fats and oils, to make hormones, such as testosterone and estrogen. Every cell in our bodies has a cell membrane composed of lipids. Every nerve is encased in a sheath of fat and would die without it. We need a protective layer of fat to keep us warm in the winter. *Triglycerides*, a type of fat, are used by muscle as a fuel. The brain and the nervous system, the immune system, the digestive system—every body part needs fats to function properly. Some vitamins, like vitamin D, are fat soluble. The intestine cannot absorb fat-soluble vitamins unless there is some fat or oil present. To move from inside the GI tract to inside your blood stream, the fat-soluble vitamins hitch a ride on fats. The list goes on and on as to the importance of fats.

But don't stop reading here and think you can go grab a bag of potato chips and a bowl of ice cream! You want to include fats

---

1. The terms fat and oil are used interchangeably in this book. In common practice, people think of oil as a liquid and fat as a solid. That is one way to look at it. But if you put oil in the refrigerator, the oil becomes a solid, and we don't start calling it a fat instead, do we? The proper medical term for a fat or an oil is lipid, which will not be used in this book.

in your diet, but they must be chosen properly. There are good fats and bad fats. The good fats include olive oil and the oils found in avocados, nuts, seeds, and fish. The bad ones include margarine and shortening, such as Crisco. A good rule of thumb is that if you read a food label and cannot pronounce one of the ingredients, that food is probably not good for you. *Partially hydrogenated vegetable oil* falls into that category.

The purpose of all the large food companies is to make money...a lot of money. The more money, the better. Their purpose is not to make foods that are healthy for you. The companies need to be able to produce a product, whether it's a cracker or a can of soup, which has a long shelf life. Those crackers you just bought yesterday were probably made a couple of months ago. Then you get home from the supermarket and put them away in the cupboard. The crackers might sit in your cupboard for a few more weeks before you finally eat them. If the oils in those crackers went rancid, the food company would lose money. In order to increase the shelf life of foods, years ago, food scientists refined a process called *hydrogenation.* This process changes the structure of that oil, so it's stable over time and does not go rancid. Have you ever noticed how if you buy a bottle of virgin olive oil, it goes rancid after a few months? Yet, if you buy a bottle of corn oil, it will last longer than a new car.

Partially hydrogenated vegetable oils, also known as *trans fats* or *trans-fatty acids*, are engineered by taking an oil, like corn oil, and subjecting it to high heat in the presence of hydrogen gas. This process changes the configuration of the chemical bonds in the oil. The oil is converted from a liquid to a solid, for example, from corn oil to margarine. The configuration is changed from *cis* to *trans*, for those of you who remember your high school chemistry. This is why partially hydrogenated vegetable oils are called trans fats or trans-fatty acids. The hydrogenation process also extends the shelf life of any food product, such as cookies or crackers, made with the hydrogenated oil. So when you finally open that package of crackers in your cupboard, they will still be fresh as a daisy. Unprocessed oils go rancid quickly, but partially hydrogenated vegetable oils don't. Bacteria aren't interested in eating partially hydrolyzed vegetable oils, and you should not be either.

Trans fats are *not* good for you. They cannot, or at least should not, be used by the body to make hormones, to make cell membranes, for brain function, or for any of those essential functions the body needs fats for. Trans fats raise the level of your LDL, which is the bad form of cholesterol, and increase your risk of heart attacks. You need to read the labels of the foods you buy. If the ingredient list contains partially hydrogenated vegetable oil or shortening or margarine, stay away from that food.

The FDA recently passed a law requiring nutrition labels to include amounts of trans fats. All the large food companies were forewarned this was going to happen and have been scrambling to remove the trans fats from your favorite foods. For the major fast-food chains, you can log onto their web sites to check the nutrition information. You'll see that most of the foods contain no, or very small amounts of, trans fats. Although the companies are not using oils that contain trans fat, the oils are still processed and refined. These processed oils don't break down after multiple uses, so the oil can be reused again and again. Batch after batch of french fries are fried in the same oil, over and over. They call this "hours of oil use" in the industry. Processed oils can be used for up to thirty hours of "oil use." You need to stay away from these fried foods. Many health food purists are going back to using butter, lard, and suet (beef fat) for frying. Our grandmothers rendered lard and suet from fatty cuts of meat, then used the fat for cooking. Little did grandma know that these fats are very stable. The oils don't break down into toxic by-products at high temperatures.

For other uses, such as salad dressings, those same health food purists stick to the tried and true: olive oil. Three of the most commonly used oils (soybean, cottonseed, and canola), are relatively new oils. They have not been used in the human diet for millennia the way that olive oil has. Corn oil, also a relatively new oil, would not be so bad for you if it was not so processed and stripped of essential fatty acids. Essential fatty acids are those that our bodies cannot manufacture; therefore, we need to get them through our diet. Real corn oil, unprocessed and cold-pressed, is the color of a rich, dark honey. The processed corn oil in the supermarket is clear, pale yellow. All the good stuff has been taken out. Essential fatty acids are removed from the oil because they are the part that turns rancid, especially when heated to high temperatures. But they are also the part of the oil that's good for your health! American ingenuity. Take a food, which started out as good for you, refine it, process it, and turn it into a killer.

If only it were so simple. There are new processed foods on the market without partially hydrogenated fats. Remember what we said earlier about the process to manufacture margarine. During the hydrogenation process, oil, such as corn oil, is subjected to heat in the presence of hydrogen gas. The process changes the configuration of the chemical bonds to produce a semi-solid fat like margarine or Crisco. Only a portion of the bonds change, thus making it *partially* hydrogenated. If the process went fully to completion, and all the bonds were changed, it would be a *fully* hydrogenated fat with the consistency of a hard wax, like a candle. It would not be suitable for cooking. You'd have to get out your cleaver to chop off a piece to melt before spreading on your bread. Some big food companies have now taken this fully hydrogenated corn oil and blended it with oil from soybeans that have been genetically modified (GM). GM soybeans were engineered to produce less of the good omega-3 linolenic oil. This oil is nicknamed *low-lin* soybean oil. This oil does not go rancid quickly because all the good stuff has been engineered out.

The oil industry proclaims that low-lin soybean oil is beneficial because it "does not oxidize easily and is relatively stable. This makes it ideal for use as a biodegradable industrial lubricant. But it turns out that *this industrial lubricant is ideal for use in processed foods* [italics mine]." [2] Industrial lubricant! Ideal for processed foods! "Honey, quick! Run out to the car, and bring back some axle grease to spread on the bagels." Some clever person (not me) came up with a new word for processed foods containing ingredients not found in nature: Frankenfoods.

You can now buy a *trans-fat-free* shortening made with fully hydrogenated corn oil blended with low-lin soybean oil. These new oil blends, formed by a process of interesterification, are called *interesterified oils*. By definition, these products are not partially hydrogenated because they are fully hydrogenated. How clever. There are no regulations requiring food companies to disclose the presence of fully hydrogenated oil in their products. You won't be able to tell if you're buying candle wax blended with industrial lubricant. These synthetic fats are not found in nature. You want to eat this stuff?

The big food companies are trying to tell us fully hydrogenated fats may actually be good for us. Are any of you old enough to remember the advertisements back in the '60s, '70s, and '80s? There was a blitz of advertising touting the benefits of margarine. It was the "healthy" alternative to butter. And don't forget about the advertising claims that corn oil was the healthy alternative to olive oil. "Switch from those 'heavy' oils to corn oil." My mom, a very fabulous Italian cook, dutifully switched from olive oil to corn oil. She certainly did not want to poison her family with olive oil! Today, we know that virgin olive oil is far superior to processed corn oil. We know margarine is bad for you.

Fool me once, shame on you. Fool me twice, shame on me. They tell us *fully* hydrogenated oils are good for us. Should we believe them now? I'd rather wait the twenty years to see if history repeats itself.

---

2. CalorieLab, "GM Soybean Oil to Aid in Reducing Trans Fat," http://calorielab .com/news/2005/12/10/gm-soybean-oil-to-aid-in-reducing-trans-fat/.

Chapter Nine

The Good, the Bad, and the Trans—Fats, That Is

So where do you begin if you want to include healthy fats in your diet every day?

The first thing is to eliminate all trans fats from your diet.

Look at the food label on the jar, bag, or box of whatever you're about to buy. There are two parts to the label. First, look at the nutrition information, which lists the calories, fats, protein, and carbohydrates in one serving. Make sure that there are no trans fats contained in that food.

Nutrition Facts

Serving Size 2/3 cup
Servings per Container about 6
Amount Per Serving
Calories 200
Fat Calories from Fat 80

Amount Per Serving	% Daily Value
Total Fat 10g	15%
Saturated Fat 4.5g	5%
Trans Fat 0g	

Cholesterol 20mg	0%
Sodium 500mg	14%
Total Carbohydrate 23g	1%
Dietary Fiber 3g	
Sugars 2g	
Protein 3g	

Next, look at the ingredient list to make sure it does not contain partially hydrogenated vegetable oil or shortening.

Ingredients: Potatoes, milk, butter, liquid soybean oil, **partially hydrogenated soybean oil**, water, salt, whey, soy lecithin, vegetable mono-and diglycerides, sodium benzoate, artificial flavors, citric acid, salt, maltodextrin, cultured dextrose, potassium sorbate, disodium pyrophosphate, sodium diacetate, xanthan gum, egg white.

Did you guess what that food was? Mashed homestyle potatoes, $5.69 for a thirty-two-ounce container (two pounds). For $5.69, you could have bought a five-pound bag of potatoes, a pound of butter, and a quart of milk and made your own mashed potatoes. Yours would not have had any trans fats or disodium pyrophosphate or sodium diacetate. Who makes mashed potatoes at home with disodium pyrophosphate? I wouldn't exactly call the store-bought tub of mashed potatoes "homestyle."

I wondered who would buy this stuff, spending $5.69 for a tub of potatoes. There were probably fifty cents worth of ingredients in there. Then, I went to a friend's house. Sitting in the refrigerator, there it was…a big plastic tub of mashed potatoes.

You, and my dear friend, need to look carefully at both the nutrition facts and the ingredient list on the food label. Notice that the tub of mashed potatoes contains partially hydrogenated soybean oil even though there aren't any trans fats listed in the nutrition facts. The large food companies are slick. If a serving size of a particular food, such as salad dressing, contains 0.5 grams of trans fats, it can be listed as *zero* grams of trans fats on the label. By making the serving size small, the label can read zero grams of trans fats. So, for example, a bottled salad dressing might list one tablespoon as the serving size with no trans fats. If you use four tablespoons of bottled salad dressing as a typical serving size, you'd be getting two grams of trans fats. You need to carefully read the labels, including the ingredient list, which would show that the food contains partially hydrogenated vegetable oil.

Some processed foods, like potato chips, will say on the label they have no trans fats. The same is true if you look at the nutrition information of your favorite fast food. Maybe they started out with no trans fats, but after getting fried at high temperatures in corn oil, they certainly don't end up as a health food. Some of the oils do get changed into trans fats after being heated to high temperatures.

Let me save you time. In order to avoid trans and other unhealthy fats, it means *no fast food!* All of it contains unhealthy fats except for the ketchup packets. Okay, I'm kidding. But fast foods are not healthy foods, and this program is for your health.

What else?

No processed peanut butter
No margarine
No packaged cookies
No candy bars (with certain exceptions described in a later chapter)
No cakes from cake mixes
No frozen waffles
No bottled salad dressing (You'll need to make your own.)
No instant soup cups
No donuts
No potato chips

Is there anything left to eat? Read on. There is plenty to eat!

The second thing, after you remove trans fats from your diet, is to make sure you include healthy fats in your diet every day. Nuts, avocados, and seeds all contain healthy fats. Eat peanuts as a snack. Buy the ones you have to shell yourself. The red, paper-like coating has nutrients that protect against heart attacks. Buy peanut butter with nothing but peanuts as an ingredient. Some peanut butters have corn syrup as well as partially hydrogenated vegetable oil; they are not on the program. When you're in the corner store looking for a snack, buy one of those small bags of nuts instead of a candy bar. If you're having a sugar craving, get a bag of trail mix with some dried fruit as well as nuts. You can even eat eggs for breakfast again! The yolks, although high in fats, may quite possibly be good for you. Eat an avocado every day, put olive oil on your salad, and include fish in your diet as often as your pocketbook allows.

The oils found in cold-water fish, such as salmon and tuna, are also essential for a healthy diet. There is overwhelming evidence that omega-3 fatty acids in the diet may decrease your risk of developing dementia and help prevent heart attacks. For example, men who have suffered a heart attack can cut their chances of having a second heart attack in half if they eat an omega-3-containing fish three times a week. All we are talking about here is a tuna sandwich on Monday, Wednesday, and Friday.

Fish living in cold ocean water have oils in their body to keep them warm and keep their blood flowing, like antifreeze. These oils are called omega-3 fatty acids[1]—omega-3 is a scientific term describing the placement of a double bond in the oil molecule—and they go a long way in the prevention of heart disease. For example, prior to the introduction of refined foods, the Inuit had no heart disease, even though their diet was very high in fat.[2] They ate a 50 percent fat diet; that is, 50 percent of the calories in their diet came from fat!

1. There are omega-3, omega-6, and omega-9 fatty acids. Omega-6 fatty acids are found in olive oil and nuts.
2. Previously called Eskimos, the people of the Far North in Canada and Greenland prefer to be called Inuit. The native people of Alaska and Siberia can still be called Eskimo, because they are not Inuit. They are Yupik, with a language and culture different from the Inuit.

(The typical American eats a 50 percent fat diet, but it's certainly not from good fats.) Virtually all of the fat in the Inuit diet came from cold-water fish and mammals containing omega-3 fatty acids.

So what can you eat to get adequate amounts of omega-3 into your diet? Well, salmon once a week or tuna, mackerel, sardines, anchovies, or mahi-mahi three times a week would satisfy the minimum requirements for omega-3 intake. Because salmon contains a greater concentration of these fish oils, you need to eat it in a smaller quantity, or less often.

Once I was giving a lecture about nutrition to a group of AIDS patients who were living in assisted-living housing because they had been homeless. One man raised his hand to ask a question. He looked like he had seen some hard times in his day. He asked if caviar contains omega-3s. Well, I was stumped. I had to go home and do a little research. For all of you caviar lovers out there, *yes*! Caviar is an excellent source of omega-3s.

Shellfish is in as well. For years, doctors have told people to avoid shellfish. Shrimp, lobster, clams, oysters, and scallops were thought to be high in cholesterol, but they are not. They have *sterols*, but not chole*sterol*. Back in the old days, the equipment used to measure cholesterol content could not differentiate between cholesterol and other sterols. Today, the equipment is much more sophisticated and can tell the difference. The sterols in shellfish do not contribute to high cholesterol. Shellfish is a good source of high-quality protein and contains omega-3 fatty acids as well as other essential nutrients.

The main concern in eating seafood so often during the week is mercury, which is particularly bad for pregnant women and children. Since mercury accumulates in your body and takes time to eliminate, the mercury you ate *one year ago* is still hanging around! If you're planning on becoming pregnant in the near future, you need to avoid mercury in your diet starting right now. Additionally, don't eat the fish's skin, and remove the line of dark meat right next to the skin, which also stores pollutants. There is more information and lists of the mercury content of many fish in appendix 6. As long as you stay vigilant about the mercury content of the fish you eat, you can include omega-3 oils in your diet in a safe way.

Fortunately, in addition to fish, there are plant-based sources of omega-3 fatty acids. Plant-based sources of omega-3 fatty acids include:

> Flaxseeds and flaxseed oil
> Walnuts and walnut oil
> Canola oil
> Wheat germ and oat germ
> Pumpkin seeds
> Hempseed and hempseed oil
>> Hemp may give you a false positive toxicology for cannabis, i.e., marijuana. Avoid hemp and hempseed oil if you work in law enforcement or if you have a job where they do routine drug screens. Additionally, the body may not convert hempseed oil into a usable form of omega-3. For now, stay away from hemp and hempseed oil until that question is resolved.
> Tofu and tempeh
>> This is why you should never buy reduced-fat soy products. The good stuff is in the plant oils.
> Dark green leafy vegetables, especially wild bitter greens

In fact, wild bitter greens are probably the second most important item in the Mediterranean diet, just behind olive oil, for health and wellness. When I was very young, our Italian grandmother lived with us. Whenever she had the chance, Grandma would go pick dandelion leaves. Yes, the weed, dandelion. Needless to say, her grandchildren were mortified. Imagine if one of our friends saw our grandmother picking weeds on the side of the road!

Flash forward forty years. My friend Dr. Judy rented a farmhouse in Virginia horse country for the summer. The lawn was full of dandelions. We called the owner to make sure he had never sprayed pesticides or herbicides on the lawn. When we got the green light, there I was, out in the backyard picking dandelions just like Grandma did. Everyone made fun of me, but at the local farmers' market, those same wild dandelion greens go for some ridiculous price like six dollars for a half a pound.

The Greek island of Crete is one of the places where the Mediterranean diet has been studied in depth. Why are the people who live on Crete so healthy? If you ask anyone who lives there, he or she will tell you that the secret to health is in the wild greens (weeds), like dandelion and purslane. Wild greens, especially purslane, are very high in omega-3 fatty acids. Almost every culture has a dark green, bitter leaf in its cuisine. Collard greens, spinach, escarole, turnip greens, beet greens, kale, Swiss chard, endive, and broccoli rabe are all on the list. The Mexicans eat salads made with verdolaga, which is another name for purslane. You could even include seaweed for those of you who like Japanese food. The Aztecs had chia seeds. Yes, the little seeds on Chia Pets are a good source of omega-3s.

You may find it odd that green leafy vegetables contain omega-3 fatty acids. Most people believe omega-3s come from fish. True, but the fish did not produce the omega-3s in the first place. These healthy fats were actually first produced by algae, which aren't really a plant, but close enough. Omega-3s help the algae stay pliable in the frigid ocean waters. Algae are eaten by the smallest fish, which are then eaten by bigger fish, so on up the food chain. The omega-3 oils become concentrated in the largest cold-water fish.

Interestingly enough, the *ratio* of omega-6s to omega-3s in our diet may be more important than the *absolute* amount of omega-3s. The traditional people of the Mediterranean eat a ratio of two to one of omega-6 to omega-3, which means they eat twice as much omega-6s as omega-3s. Our diet in America has a ratio of sixteen to one. We eat eight times too much omega-6 fats, or eight times too little omega-3s. An excess of omega-6s in the diet is associated with arthritis, allergies, asthma, osteoporosis, depression, and attention-deficient disorder. The list of diseases associated with the lack of omega-3 fatty acids keeps getting longer.

We need to take a hint from the Mediterranean people and really crank up our consumption of green leafy vegetables, not just for the omega-3s, but also for the phytonutrients and minerals. Remember to eat some oil with your green leafy vegetables. For example, eat your fresh greens with salad dressing (not a fat-free salad dressing either) or sauté the greens in olive oil. The oil helps your body absorb the fat-soluble nutrients, including the essential fatty acids.

Chapter Ten

Saturated, Polyunsaturated, and Monounsaturated Oils and Fats

You may not know the exact definition of a saturated fat versus a monounsaturated fat versus a polyunsaturated fat, but you do have some knowledge. By avoiding cholesterol in your diet, you are, without realizing it, avoiding saturated fat. When you put olive oil on your salad, you're eating a monounsaturated fat. When you eat salmon, you're taking in some polyunsaturated fats. But all oils are a mixture of fatty acids of different lengths and properties because each type of plant (and animal) has its own unique mixture. Oils, when fresh pressed from the seeds, contain a mixture of these fatty acids and traces of fat-soluble vitamins, like vitamin E. Even lard, the classic example of a saturated fat, is a mixture of fatty acids. Although 40 percent of lard is saturated fat, 45 percent (almost half) of lard is monounsaturated, just like olive oil!

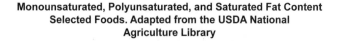

Monounsaturated, Polyunsaturated, and Saturated Fat Content Selected Foods. Adapted from the USDA National Agriculture Library

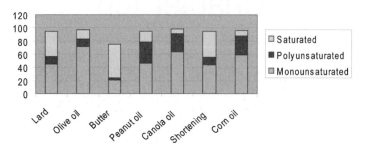

By eating these oils (mixtures of fatty acids), our body can make what it needs, except for essential fatty acids, which we cannot make ourselves. You're probably worried about adding oils back into your diet. For the last twenty years, we've heard the media blame fats for the rise in obesity in America. But did anyone ever lose weight eating low-fat cookies? Don't listen to all of that low-fat hype. Low-fat diets do not help prevent heart attacks. They do not help prevent breast cancer. They do not prevent colon cancer. They do not even seem to help anyone lose weight! During the past twenty years, in the height of the low-fat craze, Americans became bigger and bigger. Even though the sale of low-fat foods exploded, we kept gaining weight. The French have always eaten high-fat foods: lots of cheese, butter, cream, whole milk, duck, foie gras (duck liver), and eggs. And yet, the French don't get fat! The French do not die of heart attacks and strokes at the rate Americans do. This is called the French paradox. My patients still do not believe me, though, when I tell them they can add fats back to their diet. Maybe if I had some data to back me up, they'd believe me.

Recently, the Women's Health Initiative completed a large study.[1] Huge, in fact! Forty-nine thousand women were followed

---

1. B. V. Howard and others, "Low-Fat Dietary Pattern and Weight Change Over 7 Years: The Women's Health Initiative Dietary Modification Trial," *Journal of the American Medical Association* 295, no. 1 (2006): 39–49.

for eight years. Half of the group ate a low-fat diet. The other half ate a regular diet. Guess what? The low-fat group did not lose any weight. Actually, that's not completely correct. At the end of seven years, the low-fat group weighed on average one pound less than the group eating a regular diet. All that push for us to eat low-fat diet stuff was not based on reality. For those of you still stuck on the low-fat craze, realize that you cannot and should not eliminate all fats in your diet. First of all, that's impossible. All foods, including vegetables, contain a small amount of fat. Second of all, a meal with a bit of fat or oil helps to satisfy hunger. Fats take longer to digest and seem to turn off the hunger center in the brain. Have you ever noticed that when you eat a bowl of cereal with skim milk for breakfast, you're hungry again an hour later? (For a long time, I was on a low-fat diet, and I needed to eat every three hours. I also developed autoimmune thyroid disease, which I am convinced was caused by the lack of healthy oils and fats in my diet. Remember, good fats are important for a healthy immune system.) Thirdly, many vitamins are *fat-soluble*. This means they are absorbed from food only in the presence of fats. Vitamins A, D, E, and K all need fats in the diet for absorption by the body through the intestine. Fourth on the list, there are a number of essential nutrients we must get from our diets because we cannot make them ourselves: essential amino acids, essential vitamins, and *essential fatty acids*. We need to get our essential fatty acids (EFAs) from fats in our diets. EFAs are needed by our bodies to make hormones and cell membranes, to help our brains think, to keep us warm in the winter, to make hormones, and to keep our skin soft. Lastly and most importantly for you, low-fat diets just don't work and are especially bad for diabetics! There was an excellent study done in Israel.[2] Three diets were compared: Atkins, low-fat, and the Mediterranean diet. The participants, especially the women and the diabetics, did very well on the Mediterranean diet. At the end of

---

2. I. Shai and others, "Weight Loss with a Low-Carbohydrate, Mediterranean, or Low-Fat Diet," *New England Journal of Medicine* 359 (2008): 229–241.

the study, the women assigned to the low-fat diet lost no weight. None! Have I made myself clear? Low-fat diets don't work.

As you add back fats to your diet, consider the differences between monounsaturated, polyunsaturated, and saturated fats.

Monounsaturated Fats

Oils high in *mono*unsaturated fats include olive oil and peanut oil. These oils are liquid at room temperature, but get thick when refrigerated. They have *one* unsaturated bond; hence *mono*unsaturated. These oils are good for you. Avocados and nuts are also high in monounsaturated fats.

Monounsaturated fats tend to be omega-6s and omega-9s. There is a bit of debate going on in research circles as to the importance of monounsaturated fats in the diet. As we saw earlier, the ratio of omega-6 to omega-3 fats in our diet should be two to one, as opposed to the ratio of sixteen to one in the American diet. There is the camp that believes we should eat less omega-6s, and there is a lot of value in their recommendations, just as there is value in the opposing camp that recommends eating more nuts, i.e., more omega-6s. There is data that shows improvements in cholesterol levels when people add nuts to their diet. You can even buy supplements that contain omega-3, -6, and -9 in just the perfect ratio. I do not recommend buying omega-3-6-9 supplements. They would be okay if the only oils you obtained in your diet were the oils in the supplement. Since we are all eating too much in the way of omega-6, why spend good money on a supplement which contains more of what we already eat too much of?

Polyunsaturated Fats

Polyunsaturated fats are nicknamed PUFAs. Oils which contain polyunsaturated fats are also good for you. PUFAs have *two or more* unsaturated bonds. These oils are liquid at room temperature and in the refrigerator and include safflower oil, sunflower oil, soybean oil, flaxseed oil, and the oils found in cold-water fish—in other words, omega-3s. Include PUFAs in your diet every day. The question is where to get your PUFAs, because not all PUFAs are created equal. Eating fish every day is a possibility if you're a millionaire, someone else is doing the cooking, and you aren't worried about mercury. I'd wait to see long-term data on PUFAs from safflower and soybean oils. They are just too new in the human diet, unlike fish, which have been eaten by humans for thousands, if not millions, of years. Sunflower oil is another I would avoid. Studies done a few years ago showed an increase in breast and prostate cancer in animals, although the question is not settled yet. The problem may lie with PUFAs in general, especially if heated to high temperatures, and not specifically with sunflower oil.

Flaxseed oil contains omega-3s, but I would caution you against using flaxseed oil as your *only* source of PUFAs. First of all, flaxseed oil goes rancid quickly, so you need to buy it, refrigerate it, and use it quickly. Flaxseed oil has never been a staple in human diets through the millennia precisely for the reason that it goes rancid quickly. Certainly, people as far back as the Neanderthals made breads and "cakes" with whole flaxseeds, but they did not use the oil as a supplement. There were no refrigerators back then! If you want to add flax to your diet, buy the whole seeds, grind them in a small coffee grinder, and add it to your breakfast cereal. But you would have to be really gung ho about health, and have plenty of time to spare, in order to do this. You can buy a package of ground flaxseeds and store it in the freezer. They turn rancid quickly, though, and who knows how long ago the seeds were ground before they ended up in your grocery cart. If you buy the oil, make sure it's in a glass bottle. I would not trust essential fatty acids from a plastic bottle.

Saturated Fats

These fats are solid at room temperature, like butter, lard, beef fat, coconut oil, palm oil, and chicken fat. Saturated fats have been banned from every diet in the last fifty years, except Atkins. They have long been felt to be the cause of obesity, heart attacks, strokes, and cardiovascular disease. Fifteen years ago, I would have told you to ban saturated fats from your diet. To do this, you would've had to eliminate butter and cheese. You would've had to remove the skin from chicken and turkey before cooking. You would've had to bake, grill, or boil your foods instead of sautéing or frying. You would've had to remove as much fat as possible from meat before cooking, then trim any fat left after cooking, before eating the meat. Your eggs would've had to be hard-boiled instead of fried. I might have even told you to throw out the yolk—the best part!

But an appeal has been filed as the results of long-term studies become available. After many years in exile, saturated fats are being reconsidered because they may actually be innocent. The jury is still out. The data is mixed, but there are no good randomized, controlled trials that show that eating saturated fats causes heart disease! It will take scientists years of research to figure it all out. Here are quotes from two separate research articles published in prestigious medical journals. Both articles were published the very same month and came up with two separate conclusions about saturated fats.

Quote #1: "For a 5 percent lower energy intake from saturated fatty acids and a concomitant higher energy intake from polyunsaturated fatty acids, there was a significant inverse relationship between polyunsaturated fatty acids and risk of coronary events."[3] (Translation: people who ate 5 percent less saturated fat and 5 percent more PUFAs had a lower risk of heart attacks.)

Quote #2: "Higher intake of…polyunsaturated fatty acids relative to saturated fatty acids…were not significantly associated with coronary heart disease."[4] (Translation:

3. M. U. Jakobson and others, "Major Types of Dietary Fat and Risk of Coronary Heart Disease: A Pooled Analysis of 11 Cohort Studies," *American Journal of Clinical Nutrition* 89 (2009): 1425–32.
4. A. Mente and others, "A Systemic Review of the Evidence Supporting a Causal Link Between Dietary Factors and Coronary Heart Disease," *Archives of Internal Medicine* 169, no. 7 (2009): 659–669.

people who ate less saturated fat but more PUFAs did not have a lower risk of heart attacks.)

So which is correct? Those two articles may have disagreed on the role of saturated fat, but they agreed on one important point. A diet high in starches and sweets leads you down the road to heart disease. How many of you eat two donuts for breakfast instead of two eggs because of the cholesterol in the yolk? You are not doing your body a favor. It's far better to eat the eggs and skip the donuts.

Plus, your cholesterol level isn't the only thing determining your risk of having a heart attack. Remember our friends, the Inuit, who ate a diet in which 50 percent of the calories came from fat. In the original study, the Inuit were compared to people living in Denmark. When cholesterol levels were measured in their blood, the numbers for the Inuit and the Danes were exactly the same. But the Inuit had far fewer heart attacks. How could this be? The numbers that came back from the lab didn't mean a thing! There is more to a heart attack than just cholesterol.

Moderate amounts of saturated fat in the context of an otherwise healthy diet does not raise LDL. On the other hand, if all your fat calories are coming from saturated fats, and all of your carbohydrate calories are coming from sweets and starches, your LDL (bad) cholesterol goes through the roof, and your HDL (good) cholesterol goes down the drain. This kind of diet slows your mind, makes you gain weight, and leads you down the road to diabetes. Saturated fats, sweets, and starches are a recipe for disaster. It's really quite easy to get all of your fat calories from saturated fat and all of your carbohydrate calories from sweets and starches. It's called the American diet.

The bottom line is, go ahead. Add fats and oils to your diet. Make sure you eat mono- and polyunsaturated fats. Use olive oil on your salad. Eat nuts as a snack, and eat fish at least three times a week. Add an avocado to your salad as often as you like, every day even, if it makes you happy. Eat a dark green leafy vegetable every single day because they too contain omega-3s.

If you love butter and cheese, go ahead and eat them, but in moderation. Saturated fats are not the enemy, but you do need to use them in moderation because they are high in calories. Remember, calories count. Whether the fat in your diet is coming from fried pork rinds or from olive oil, it's a high-calorie food and can pack on the pounds if you overdo it.

Chapter Eleven

HFCS is Not a Bank

High fructose corn syrup, abbreviated HFCS, is a processed food product made from, no surprise, corn. Fructose is a naturally occurring sugar found in fruit. Since fruit is good for you, HFCS should be really good for you too. Right? Wrong! HFCS is another additive to be avoided completely.

In real fruit, fructose is bound to fiber and complex carbohydrates. The fiber helps keep your colon moving and the complexity of the carbohydrates does not dump a load of sugar into your stomach all at once. Eating an orange does not give you a sugar high the way a candy bar does. Most importantly, compared to HFCS, there is only a small amount of fructose in fruit. Fruit also contains vitamins, minerals, and *phytochemicals*, although phyto*nutrients* is probably a better term. Although phytonutrients cannot be classified as vitamins or minerals, they are antioxidants and are essential for health.

HFCS is in almost every processed food. And if a processed food does not have HFCS, it probably contains corn in some form or another. Corn is cheap. HFCS is cheap. The government makes sure it stays that way through farm subsidies. Farm subsidies would be great if they were helping the family farms that have been the backbone of American agriculture for generations. But the farm subsidies aren't helping these hardworking farmers; they are only helping the big food companies. These subsidies keep the price of corn low, so HFCS stays cheap, and the food companies can keep making soda and corn oil and Count Chocula cereal.

HFCS is used in soft drinks, candies, cookies, and breakfast cereals. You even find it in foods you would never imagine: Frozen meatloaf! Ketchup! Peanut butter! The bottom line is that you cannot eat or drink anything that contains HFCS if you want to lose weight, if you are diabetic or prediabetic, or if you simply want to be in the best shape of your life. Sodas and sweets seem to be especially efficient at contributing to belly fat.

For many people, the first step toward health is to stop drinking soda. Besides HFCS, soda is full of chemicals. If you're already overweight and diabetes runs in your family, drinking soda is one way to make sure you'll develop diabetes too. There was a patient at our clinic who was obese, wheelchair-bound, and young (only thirty-nine years old). Twenty years of adult-onset diabetes had finally damaged the nerves in her feet, a condition called *peripheral neuropathy,* to the point where she couldn't even stand up. This woman weighed 275 pounds, but she insisted she ate very little, so I asked her to keep a food log. On her log, she wrote everything she ate or drank for three days. Sure enough, she did eat very little: three saltine crackers for breakfast, one slice of American cheese for lunch, and one chicken leg for dinner. That's less than 400 calories. Even supermodels eat more than that. Where were all the extra calories coming from for her? Soda! She was drinking two two-liter bottles of cola every day. That's *2,000* calories. This woman was diabetic—what was she thinking?

This is not negotiable.

No soda.

Period.

But my patients are clever. Before I caught on, I would tell my patients to stop drinking soda. They would replace the soda with endless glasses of fruit juice, sweetened iced tea, or Kool-Aid. Now I've learned my lesson, and I run through the whole list every time:

> No soda (No ginger ale either! Ginger ale is soda too)
> No fruit juice (too high in calories and sugars)
> No iced tea
> No beer or alcohol (except for an occasional glass of wine with a meal, or an occasional beer at a barbeque on a hot summer day)
> No Kool-Aid
> No Gatorade or sports drinks (unless you have just finished a five-mile run)

Even after I go through this whole list, someone finds something sweet to drink that I forgot to mention. One diabetic patient stopped drinking soda. He had not switched to iced tea or fruit juice or Kool-Aid. But he got me. He switched to Chocolate Yoo-hoo. I was very impressed at how resourceful he was. No matter what crazy soda substitute you can dream up, it's not on the program if it's sweetened with sugar or high fructose corn syrup.

My patients ask about diet soda. This program is about health. Diet soda is artificially flavored and artificially sweetened with chemicals. Stay away from diet soda. Not only that, but new research shows that diet soda is not good for diabetics; it may even contribute to the development of diabetes! This is extraordinary. In some studies, people who drank diet soda were more likely to develop diabetes than the non-soda drinkers. The body's response to sugar and sweets is more complicated than we ever imagined. It may be that diet soda turns on hunger signals in the body. The body sends a signal to the brain. "Feed me!" You end up eating more in the long run. Why drink this stuff?

People always want me to tell them what to drink instead of soda or diet soda. Drink water! Water is free from the tap, so you don't need to lug it home from the supermarket. Folklore tells us to drink two liters of water, or eight glasses, a day. New scientific research has shown that it may not be necessary to drink that much water. On the other hand, if you're exercising every day, and you're losing weight, you may need eight, or more, glasses of water a day. Go by how you feel; when you're thirsty, drink water.

Ah, if it only were that simple. The same way a smoker craves a cigarette, diabetics actually crave sweets. All the diabetic or predia-betic patients in my practice have an insatiable craving for sweets. So, just as no one can resist the urge to scratch an itch, diabetics cannot resist the urge to drink something sweet. The only way to break the vicious cycle is to completely *stop* all sweets, cold turkey. This means quitting all soda, juice, iced tea, beer, sports drinks, and so on.

Besides sweetened soft drinks, there is a whole list of HFCS-containing foods to avoid. You need to read the food labels, but here is a short list to start with:

> Breakfast cereals (with very few exceptions)
> Processed peanut butter
> Bottled salad dressing
> Karo syrup
> Frozen dinners
> Most canned soups
> Ketchup (Find a brand that does not have HFCS. Organic ketchup does not have HFCS, and has five times more antioxidants.)
> Some jarred tomato sauces

My friend Kim, who is Dr. Judy's sister, tells a story about a birthday cake she bought at a supermarket. It had hot pink flowers and bright yellow decorations. You know the kind of sheet cakes I'm talking about. Those flowers and decorations are made out of Karo syrup and shortening. One of the kids was running around outside with her piece of cake. Some of the flower decorations fell off the cake and onto the driveway of the house. Kim decided to let the hot pink flowers and yellow ribbons sit there in the driveway. She wanted to see how long they would take to dissolve. Well, they sat there for weeks, just little blobs of hot pink and bright yellow color in the driveway. They lasted through days of rain and days of blazing sunshine. The ants avoided those little blobs of color. Which brings us to another good rule of thumb: if the bugs don't want to eat it, neither should you.

Chapter Twelve

"Rice and Beans" Is Not a Vegetable

L et's review the changes you have made so far.

1. You have stopped drinking soda, juice, or other sweet drinks.

2. You put your body on a schedule and are eating three meals and two small snacks every day.

3. You started exercising.

4. You have stopped eating fast food and have cut out all trans fats.

5. You have added back some healthy fats to your diet, especially omega-3 fatty acids.

6. You cut out all foods with HFCS.

That's pretty darn good. Congratulations! What's next? *Eat your fruits and vegetables.*

First, we need to define fruits and vegetables. My friend, Dr. Judy, tells a story about the time she took a cross-country car trip and stopped into a Sonic drive-in. She asked if they had any vegetables.

"Fried cheese sticks," was the reply. Fried cheese sticks are not a vegetable. Are we clear on that? Or how about the time Dr. Judy's sister, Kim, was babysitting a friend's obese eight-year-old daughter? The girl wanted a piece of cake for breakfast. Kim asked the little girl to have a piece of fruit instead. "I already had a strawberry and a cherry and an orange," the girl said. Well, Kim knew something was wrong because not one piece of fruit was missing from the fruit bowl. Turns out the little girl had eaten Starbursts: strawberry-, cherry-, and orange-flavored Starbursts. Strawberry Starbursts are not a fruit. Or what about the story Dr. Judy tells of a mom with her cute little toddler at a clinic in Philadelphia. The mom pulled a can of orange soda out of her bag, popped the top, and filled the baby's bottle. "The baby is thirsty. Let me give her some juice." Orange soda is not juice. "Rice and beans" is not a vegetable. Are we all on the same page?

Vegetables include all of your green leafy vegetables (spinach) and nonleafy vegetables (cauliflower). You could include roots in your vegetable list (potatoes, yucca), but since they are starchy, we won't be eating them often. Then there is the argument as to whether zucchini is a fruit or a vegetable. Technically, vegetables like tomatoes and zucchini are fruits, but I don't think that matters much for our purposes here.

Now that we know what a vegetable is, we need to eat more of them. Several years ago, the National Cancer Institute (NCI) began a program called "Five-a-Day," referring to a diet that included five servings of fruits and vegetables every day. This program was begun due to the enormous amount of scientific evidence that a diet with lots of vegetables and fruits reduces the risk of heart disease and some cancers. As a matter of fact, for people with hypertension, the recommendation is to eat *ten* servings of fruit and vegetables a day. The antioxidants contained in fruits and vegetables protect the heart from the effects of an elevated blood pressure. Every day, I pick up one of the scientific journals and see the results of yet another study showing how fruits and vegetables in the diet prevent Alzheimer's disease, lower the risk of strokes, or prevent blindness from macular degeneration. The list goes on and on.

The five-a-day program is simple, yet only one-third of adults meet the NCI recommendation. The statistics for children are even more dismal. Only one-fifth of children meet the recommendation of eating five servings of fruits and vegetables per day. When the government first compiled the data, the statistics were even worse, even though they took into account the soggy pieces of iceberg lettuce and pickle slices on fast-food hamburgers, and the little bits of raisins in some breakfast cereals. So they went back and recalculated the numbers a second time, but included ketchup and french fries as vegetables, and thus, they came up with the current statistics. The USDA only had a budget of one million dollars to publicize the importance of fruits and vegetables. Compare that to the fifty-seven million dollars McDonald's spent in one year on advertising *just geared to Hispanics alone.*

If you're in the habit of eating a bagel for breakfast, a hamburger and fries for lunch, and rice and beans for dinner, you're not eating any vegetables at all. How is it possible to eat five to ten servings of fruits and vegetables each and every day, day in and day out, for the rest of your life? Five servings a day! Ten servings a day! A daunting task! It's not as hard as you think.

First, we need to define a serving size for fruits and vegetables. My favorite story from the clinic is about a mother with an obese child. He was twelve years old and weighed 170 pounds, so the physician assistant was telling the mother to encourage healthy-eating habits in her son. The mother replied that she was doing just that. She wants him to eat his vegetables, so when they go to McDonald's, she gets a Big Mac for him. "It has lettuce, onions, and a pickle on it." One piece of soggy lettuce, chopped onions, and a pickle slice: they do not count for much.

A serving size is considered:

> 1 cup green leafy vegetable uncooked (lettuce and salad greens)

½ cup green leafy vegetable cooked (kale, spinach, etc.)
½ cup nonleafy vegetable (cauliflower, broccoli, carrots, etc.)
1 medium fruit or ½ cup cut-up fruit
¼ cup dried fruit
6 ounces of fruit juice (apple juice, orange juice, etc.)

Start by making small substitutions. Instead of a piece of cake or some cookies for your three o'clock snack, get a banana and an orange. Better yet, have a piece of chicken and an orange, or a piece of cheese and an apple. Especially if you're diabetic, you need a bit of protein with your snacks.

Have juice instead of a soda, but there is a word of caution about juice. You cannot drink a big sixty-ounce bottle of apple juice and think that you've done a great job getting your ten servings of fruits and vegetables for the day. Juices have calories, and if you're overweight, you cannot drink endless glasses of juice. You can have juice, but a small amount.

A few years ago, I was giving a lecture in East Harlem about ways to eat ten servings of fruits and vegetables every day. I polled the audience to see if anyone actually did. There was a woman in her seventies; she looked fabulous. She could have passed for fifty-nine instead of seventy-six. She ate her ten servings every day. She ate spinach, lemons, mangos—just lots of good healthy food. There was another person in the audience who claimed that he too ate his ten servings of fruits and vegetables every day. Even more than ten servings, he claimed. Well, this young man was the size of a Mack truck, a big, blubbery guy. He was short and round. The audience all turned around to stare. They could not believe it! He got his ten servings all right, from apple juice. He drank big bottles of apple juice all day. With 110 calories in each eight-ounce glass, he was taking in close to 1,000 calories from apple juice alone. No wonder why he was so round. You cannot get all ten of your servings of fruits and vegetables from fruit juice alone. Fruit juices are a concentrated source of sugars and will really pack on the pounds if you're not careful. When you are trying to increase your intake of fruits and vegetables, limit your fruit juices to *one* serving a day.

If you really crave sweet drinks, make a pitcher of homemade lemonade, keep it in the refrigerator, and grab a glass of lemonade instead of a soda. Check this out: the nutrition label for a bottle of store-bought lemonade made with real fruit juice.

Nutrition Facts
Serving Size 8 fl oz (240 mL)
Servings Per Container 2.5
Amount Per Serving
Calories 110

CONTAINS: WATER, HIGH FRUCTOSE CORN SYRUP, LEMON JUICE FROM CONCENTRATE, CITRIC ACID, NATURAL FLAVORS, PRESERVATIVES, SODIUM CHLORIDE, ASCORBIC ACID (VITAMIN C), YELLOW DYE 6.

In little letters on the back of the bottle are the words "contains less than 3% juice." Can you read those little letters? If not, here they are again, "CONTAINS LESS THAN 3% JUICE."

Someone paid one dollar for this bottle of high fructose corn syrup with water and 3 percent juice. For a dollar, you could have made a pitcher of lemonade instead! Lemonade you make at home is an exception to the juice rule. Squeeze one or two lemons, add water and brown sugar, and you have a delicious and refreshing glass of lemon juice. You can have lots of lemonade as long as you do not go crazy with the sweeteners.

After you make small changes (fruit instead of a piece of cake, small glass of juice instead of soda), it's time to get serious. Start making salads for lunch. Have vegetables every single night with dinner. A friend of mine has a great system. She is really busy—full-time job, three children, two stepchildren, a big house, and a husband who needs attention. She puts out a platter of raw vegetables with a dip before dinner. The kids snack on carrots, broccoli, celery, and tomatoes, and they love it. You should see her children. They are the picture of health and happiness.

So in order to get ten servings of fruits and vegetables in a day, you could:

Breakfast: Put 1 cup of fruit into a breakfast smoothie (two servings). Since blueberries may help the brain and nervous system stay young, use 1½ cups of frozen blueberries in your smoothie, which counts as three servings of fruit. (See the recipe section for a power-packed blueberry shake.)

Lunch: A salad with 3 cups of lettuce and a can of tuna will give you three servings of vegetables, and a dose of omega-3s too. Get a can of V8 juice instead of a soda for another two servings of fruits and vegetables. If you use radicchio, which is that dark red, small round head of lettuce, you get an additional benefit of lots of beta-carotene and lots of phytonutrients. It has a slightly bitter taste, but it's oh so good for you. Though it's a bit expensive, one head goes a long way. It's worth trying it once.

Three o'clock snack: An orange, with a piece of cheese or grilled chicken, will give you another serving of a fruit. If it's too much trouble to pack a snack, buy a snack bag of dried fruits and nuts.

Dinner: A cup of sautéed spinach or a bowl of salad would give you two servings of vegetables. Make your dessert a bowl of grapes or melon slices for your last one to two servings.

There you have it. You can eat even more than ten servings of fruits and vegetables just by making a few changes. In addition, there are powdered fruit and vegetable extracts on the market. Appendix 7 describes these green powders in more detail. One scoop is the equivalent of five servings of vegetables. If you put one scoop into your breakfast shake every morning, along with your frozen fruit, by ten in the morning you could have seven or eight servings of fruits and vegetables. You could start your day with a boost of energy instead of a brain fog.

When choosing your fruits and vegetables, pick vine ripened whenever possible. Phytonutrients do not have time to develop in produce harvested too early, but they are part of the produce we want. They are cancer-fighting, cardio-protective, antiaging antioxidants. Here in America, fruits and vegetables are picked long before they are ripe. They ship better that way. Those of you who are old enough may remember back when fruit tasted like fruit, not like cardboard. Some of my patients, as the first step in this program, start adding salads to their diet. They buy iceberg lettuce and tomatoes. Well, it's no surprise that they hate salads. Iceberg lettuce was bred to ship well. It was not bred to taste good. The same is true for tomatoes. Don't even bother buying tomatoes in the supermarket. Red Styrofoam. The same is true for strawberries.

Years back, I was in France for a medical conference and stopped into a produce market to pick up some fruit. From the doorway, I could see a fruit stand on the other side of the market with strawberries piled up. Even from clear across the market, the strawberries didn't look that appealing. They were small and misshaped, nothing like those big perfect specimens we have in America. The thought wasn't half-formed in my mind when I was hit with the overwhelming perfume of strawberries—clear across from the other side of the market. Now *these* were strawberries! They were unlike any strawberry you've ever eaten in America. You could say the same about the peaches, melons, figs, or any other locally grown fruit or vegetable. In Europe, they have a very different system for growing and distributing farm products. Foods are more likely to be grown locally, so they can be picked ripe and transported from the farm to the consumer faster. You could argue that the Europeans have a less efficient system than ours. Perhaps. On the other hand, you could argue that their system is *more* efficient. They use less fertilizer, and they are not shipping strawberries two thousand miles by truck, using precious gasoline. Most importantly, maybe the European system is more efficient because their food is healthier.

Everybody asks if organic is better. There is a range of organic. It's expensive to become certified, so some traditional farmers with a small herd of cows might not be certified. These cows are moved from field to field, allowing the animals to exercise and eat a variety of grasses and herbs. On the other hand, some big food companies are certified organic. The cows are fed organic grain but never see the light of day. These animals live in crowded feedlots, standing (not walking because the lots are so crowded) around in their own poop. It's organic, but not exactly what you have in mind when you want to buy healthy organic meat.

Don't get me wrong. Organic is important, whether certified or not, poop notwithstanding! Some of the pesticides and herbicides used to grow nonorganic produce are very closely related in chemical structure to human hormones. They can turn off, or worse yet, turn on our hormone receptors. These chemicals are called *endocrine disruptors* or *endocrine mimics*. This is not a good thing, especially for children. Foods your children eat or drink a lot of, milk for example, might be a good idea to buy organic. For more information on organic vegetables, there is a short list in appendix 1. Since organic foods are expensive, you might need to pick and choose where to spend your precious food dollars.

If you're on a budget, don't worry about organic. Don't worry about free range. There are a lot of people out there trying to change the way America grows food. Someday we may see a revolution, so everyone can eat healthy nutritious food from plants grown without pesticides and from animals eating a diet that nature intended for them to eat. For now, just concentrate on eating your fruits and vegetables.

Chapter Thirteen

Wine, Chocolate, Lemons, and Parsley

What in the world do wine, chocolate, lemons, and parsley have in common? Antioxidants! All these foods are good for you and contain large amounts of antioxidants.

It's tough to define antioxidants in layman's terms. A good example of antioxidants can be seen when someone is making apple pie. As the apple is cut, the edges turn brown. They are *oxidizing*. If you sprinkle the cut side of the apple with lemon juice, it prevents the discoloration. The lemon juice prevented oxidation of the apple.

An antioxidant is a chemical or a molecule that protects the body from damage caused by oxidation or free radicals. No, we are not talking about the Black Panthers. The body is truly like an engine, burning fuel for energy. Just like a fire in a furnace produces sparks, your body's metabolism produces free radicals. These sparks shoot out and damage anything they hit. The body, an amazing chemical factory, uses antioxidants to attract and soak up the sparks so they don't damage the delicate machinery inside cells. Antioxidants prevent rust, so to speak. In the body, antioxidants help keep us young.

People who have the highest levels of antioxidants in their blood are less likely to suffer from heart disease, strokes, blindness, dementia, kidney disease, and the list goes on. Plenty of antioxidants in the diet may help prevent certain kinds of cancer and autoimmune disease. Best of all, antioxidants keep us feeling great and looking young.

Some people need more antioxidants than others. Athletes need more than couch potatoes. The elderly need more than the young. People with chronic diseases, like rheumatoid arthritis, need more than the average person without a chronic disease. If you're on a diet and losing weight, you really need to ramp up your intake of antioxidants. If you have diabetes, you need to ramp up your intake of foods containing antioxidants as well. Diabetics produce free radicals faster than Hollywood pumps out silly movies.

Where do you find antioxidants? Fruits, vegetables, nuts, and beans are full of antioxidants. You could buy pills at the health food store, but you're far better off when your antioxidants are from real food. Scientists have been trying for years to extract the magic ingredient from vegetables and put it into a pill. There have been innumerable studies in which one group of people was given a vitamin or antioxidant, and another group was not. A couple of studies have shown a small benefit from taking vitamin supplements; however, the vast majority of studies have shown no benefit. Even worse, in some studies, the people who took the antioxidant pills did worse than the group who did not get the pills! There is nothing like the real deal: good, healthy fruits and vegetables.

So antioxidants are what parsley, lemons, chocolate, and red wine all have in common. For those of you who are interested, you could log on to the USDA web site. There are lists of the antioxidant contents of foods. Some foods are off-the-chart good for you: parsley, beets, beans, lentils, dark green leafy vegetables (kale, spinach, Swiss chard, collard greens), and chocolate. This is the Mediterranean diet and the French paradox you keep hearing about. The newspapers keep harping on the red wine. The media would lead you to believe that the Italians live longer because they drink red wine. The French eat bread, butter, foie gras, and cheese but don't get fat because they drink red wine. The Greeks don't die of heart attacks because they drink red wine. That's only half the story. Our friends in the Mediterranean do drink wine, yes, and lots of it. But for Europeans, wine is always part of a meal. Our French friends eat butter and cheese, yes, but in moderation. The cheese is from animals eating wild greens out in the pasture, as opposed to corn in a feedlot in the Midwest. Europeans eat bread, yes, but good, old-fashioned, fresh-baked crusty French or Italian bread. They are not eating mushy white bread from a plastic bag. When they do eat bread, they eat one piece, not the whole loaf. The people of the Mediterranean eat less meat, and not every day. When they do eat meat, it's often lamb, especially in Greece and southern Italy. Lamb has another healthy fat called CLA, which may prevent certain kinds of cancer. Lentils and beans are substituted for meat at many meals. HFCS is only found in imported American soda, and sugary desserts are a treat, not a meal. Europeans eat loads of vegetables and cook with garlic and olive oil. They get plenty of exercise, and they sure don't eat as much as we do.

Dessert for Europeans might be a small piece of dark chocolate. More likely, dessert consists of beautiful ripe fruits with some nuts. There is something important about nuts and the Mediterranean diet. It may actually be the nuts that are protecting the heart. Walnuts lower levels of bad cholesterol, and almonds may do the same. This reminds me of how we grew up, before my family became completely Americanized. Dessert was a bowl of fruit and a basket of nuts. These nuts were still in the shells. It was work to crack the shells and pick out the nut inside. There was no way you could mindlessly eat 1,000 calories worth of walnuts, unless you wanted to sit there until midnight with the nutcracker.

So how do we begin to eat like the French or the Italians or the Spanish or the Greeks or any Mediterranean culture?

Let's start with the wine. The ingredients in red wine that make your mouth pucker are antioxidants. You could drink a glass of red wine, even two glasses, every night with dinner. A good recommendation for men perhaps, but it's not a good recommendation for women. More than two alcoholic drinks a week may increase the risk of breast cancer in women. At most, have a small glass of red wine with dinner on Friday and Saturday nights. The Europeans always drink their wine with a meal. Always!

If you're diabetic, you should avoid wine, or any alcohol for that matter. If you're not diabetic but hate wine, you could have a small glass of grape juice instead. Juice still has antioxidants, though not as much. If you hate red wine but like white wine, go ahead. White wine has fewer antioxidants, twenty times less in fact, but they are still there. Wine, like everything else in life, should be done in moderation. If you need to lose weight, wine has calories, and you need to watch your intake. Remember, moderation!

Chocolate is probably going to be your favorite part of increasing your intake of antioxidants. Scientific studies have shown that people with the highest intake of cocoa have fewer heart attacks. Cocoa even lowers blood pressure! Yes, in some controlled scientific studies, eating chocolate every day, even just a little bit, lowers blood pressure.[1] Don't run for the chocolate ice cream yet, though. Most of the chocolate in the supermarket or the corner bodega is processed to the point where all of the antioxidants are destroyed. The chocolate you buy must be dark chocolate, not milk chocolate. Look at the ingredient list before you buy a bar. If partially hydrogenated vegetable oil is one of the ingredients, that chocolate bar is not on the program. If high fructose corn syrup is one of the ingredients, that chocolate bar is not on the program. Let me save you time. Most of the candy bars at the corner bodega are not

---

1. B. Buijsse and others, "Cocoa Intake, Blood Pressure, and Cardiovascular Mortality: The Zutphen Elderly Study," *Archives of Internal Medicine* 166 (2006): 411–417.

on the program. All the chocolate syrups you pour from a plastic bottle are not on the program. Most of the chocolate ice creams in the supermarket are not on the program.

You need to seek out items like CocoaVia candy bars from Mars. The cocoa in CocoaVia is specially processed so the antioxidants are not destroyed. They are a little difficult to find, but some large drugstores sell them, or you could buy them over the Internet. Keep your eyes open for these delicious little chocolate bars. Dove also has a dark chocolate candy bar I have just started seeing in the corner stores. Dove and CocoaVia are both from the Mars company, which has spent many years and many millions of dollars researching the health benefits of cocoa. Mars also just came out with a chocolate drink called CocoaPro. I suspect we will be seeing more chocolate bars and drinks from Mars as they continue their research and product development.

Chocolate is a treat, not a meal replacement. You cannot have two candy bars as your three o'clock snack, and tell your friends it's okay because you read it here. A small piece of dark chocolate, once a day or every other day, is a special treat. Eat it slowly, and enjoy it. You didn't become overweight because you do things in moderation. Eat chocolate in moderation and enjoy it.

Lemons, unlike chocolate, you can go overboard with. Lemons are full of vitamins, antioxidants, and phytochemicals. Use them for their antibacterial, anticancer, antiarthritis, and antiaging effects. They are cheap and available in every supermarket across America. Back in the 1870s in the Wild West, they were coveted and prized for their health benefits, so they sold for a dollar a lemon! That would be fifteen to twenty dollars today. There is something interesting about the antioxidants in lemons. Limonin, one of the antioxidants in lemons, has a very long half-life, which means it stays in your bloodstream a long time. This is a good thing; it means the antioxidant effect lasts long after you take your last sip of lemonade. All those generations of grandmothers who gave children lemon with honey for a cold knew what they were doing.

For a delicious, powerhouse soda substitute, squeeze two lemons and add eight ounces of cold water and ice. You'll need to sweeten the lemonade. It's your choice whether to use a *small* amount of sugar or an artificial sweetener. However, since artificial sweeteners and refined sugar are not good for you, a good compromise is to use a *small* amount of brown sugar. Brown sugar is white sugar with some molasses added back in.

Molasses has all sorts of minerals like magnesium and manganese and is high in antioxidants. Molasses is the good part of the sugar cane that is extracted during the sugar-making process and is then sold back to you separately. If you can stand to use molasses to sweeten your lemonade, by all means, go ahead. Using molasses as the sweetener for your lemonade makes the lemonade taste like iced tea.

If you have the money, you can buy real brown sugar from an organic supermarket. These natural brown sugars never had the molasses taken out. When the sugar cane juice is collected and boiled down, these natural brown sugars are collected. They are never refined and never bleached. Be forewarned, these natural brown sugars are expensive.

Another natural sweetener is stevia. It's the ground-up leaves of the stevia plant. Some patients are gung ho about their quest for health and buy stevia to use as a sweetener. You could try a bit of stevia as the sweetener for your lemonade, but don't spend a lot of money for a big container—you may not like it. Some say it has a slightly bitter edge to it. Others say it just tastes weird.

You could also use honey to sweeten your lemonade, but that is an expensive proposition. Another natural sweetener out there is agave, the naturally sweet liquid from the agave plant, which grows in Central America and the southwestern United States. It's very sweet and has the added benefit of having a low glycemic index, so it will not spike your blood sugar. However, agave will also cost you quite a bit of change.

No matter what you use as your sweetener—Splenda, Sweet'N Low, NutraSweet (I do not recommend any artificial sweeteners), white sugar, brown sugar, molasses, honey, or agave—go easy. Remember what I wrote in the HFCS chapter. You really crave sweets and need to break the addiction. If you're a soda drinker or if you have a big sweet tooth, you'll be tempted to really pour it on. Your taste buds have gotten used to tasting nothing but the sugar. Cut back on the sweeteners and really taste the lemon. Lemonade is supposed to pucker your mouth. That's part of the enjoyment and fun of drinking lemonade.

Squeezing lemons may be too time-consuming for those of you with children, a job, and a household to manage. Minute Maid sells bottles of frozen lemon juice. Each bottle contains the juice of seven lemons and costs around two or three dollars. It's not as good as the real deal made from fresh-squeezed lemons, but it's pretty close. You can have a pitcher of homemade lemonade in your refrigerator all the time without a lot of fuss and bother. Stay away from commercially prepared lemonade and frozen lemonade. They are overly sweet and contain very little lemon juice.

Your next mission on the quest for antioxidants is parsley. Any deep dark green leafy vegetable with a slightly bitter taste fits the bill. It seems as though the more bitter the vegetable, the better it is for you. There is no getting around it: these bitter, dark green leafy vegetables are a pain in the neck to clean. Almost all of them have curly leaves and need to be washed two, three, or even four or five times to rinse off all the soil and sand. Sometimes I think you can rate how healthy a particular green is for you by how long it takes to wash. Dandelion and escarole take the longest to wash, so they must be the best for you. You can minimize your work by planning ahead and being organized. If you know you want to make Swiss chard for example, fill your sink with water. Lay the greens on top and go do something else for fifteen minutes. The sand and soil will fall to the bottom of the sink. Come back and lift out the Swiss chard carefully so as not to stir up the sand from the bottom of the sink. Wash off the sand from the bottom of the sink, and do it again. Go do something else for fifteen minutes, come back, and do it again. Keep doing it until you cannot feel any sand on the bottom of the sink.

This method assumes your sink is clean in the first place. It assumes your counters aren't cluttered with dirty dishes. It assumes you started to think about cooking Swiss chard for dinner an hour before dinnertime, and not ten minutes before. Plan ahead, and be organized. Planning and organization will help you become a great cook. And so, the next chapter is about organization.

Chapter Fourteen

Get Organized!

The quest for organization has two parts: short-term organization and long-term organization.

Short-Term Organization

Short-term organization is the day-to-day planning to maximize your success.

Pack your lunch, snacks, and a bottle of water to take with you to work. If you don't have a refrigerator at work, buy an insulated bag and ice packs.

If your mornings are hectic, *plan and pack your food the night before*. Make mental notes of the number of calories. You may not be counting calories, but you do need to make sure your breakfast will hold you until lunchtime. Make mental notes of what you're going to eat, and when you're going to eat it. If you don't plan, you'll end up eating too much or too little. Make sure you're never stranded on the subway or in the car at 6:00 p.m., starving. That's when you're tempted to stop at a fast-food restaurant for a quick cheeseburger.

Keep a protein bar, Balance Bar, or Zone Bar in your purse, your briefcase, or the glove compartment of your car. Better than a bar, make little bags of nuts and dried fruit. Make sure you have one packed before you leave the house.

There is no excuse for poor planning. If you leave the house at 6:00 a.m. and don't get home until 7:00 p.m., make sure you have packed breakfast, lunch, and at least two snacks.

Long-Term Organization

This is the planning you do for the week or the month.

Plan your exercise strategy for the week. If you belong to a gym, check the aerobics schedule to plan the classes you'll take over the next week. Make exercise dates with friends. Plan your exercise the way you would plan a movie or dinner date. You could even make a spa experience out of it! Meet a couple of your friends at the gym on a Friday evening after work. Exercise, hang out, lay in the sauna and sweat, take a leisurely shower, and then slather yourself in body oil. Afterward, go out for a healthy dinner. You'll be in heaven.

Maybe you don't belong to a gym. Some gyms will let you buy a day pass. For not much more money than the cost of the movies, you'll have a far better, self-fulfilling experience. Spoil yourself! If money is an issue, make your own gym-spa party. Invite friends over. Have one person bring over an exercise DVD, and another can bring over massage oil. Someone else can bring the crudités, and another friend can bring grilled chicken. Exercise to the tape together, eat a healthy dinner, and then give each other upper back massages. You'll have a blast.

Plan your food for the week, and then go to the grocery store pre-pared. Sit down and plan your food for the week. I don't mean for you to sit down and say, "I will eat three rice cakes at exactly 3:00 p.m. on Thursday." No, but you do need to have enough food in the house so you can pack a lunch and snack every day to bring to work.

Food is expensive. There are staples you'll need; however, you cannot buy them all at once. Spread out buying the staples: some this week and others next week. Know exactly what you'll be cooking over the next few days. Buy only what you need. Buy less than you need. Supermarkets will not fall off the face of the earth. You can always go back to pick up what you missed. It's better than wasting money on food that will rot in your refrigerator because you bought too much in the first place.

Buy Staples for the Kitchen

Kitchen staples, in addition to those listed below, include frozen vegetables and canned beans so that you can throw together a healthy meal in a pinch.

Balsamic Vinegar

Decent balsamic vinegar is very expensive. The stuff you buy in the supermarket for two or three dollars a bottle is awful, simply awful. The cheap supermarket balsamic vinegar has a bit of balsamic vinegar in it, but mostly, it's red wine vinegar, caramel coloring, and flavorings.

Real balsamic vinegar has the word *tradizionale* in the title, for example, "Aceto Balsamico Tradizionale di Reggio Emilia." Translated, that means "traditional balsamic vinegar of the Emilia region." This vinegar is made from grapes and aged in barrels. Like fine wine, it's very expensive.

You can buy very good balsamic vinegar without tradizionale in the title. The tradizionale title can only be used on balsamic vinegars from two regions of Italy; the name is protected by law. It's the same for a Vidalia onion, which only comes from Georgia. The same onion grown in North Carolina would be called a sweet onion, never a Vidalia onion. A nontradizionale balsamic vinegar is made in the same way as a tradizionale one, from grapes and aged in barrels, but it's not from one of the two designated regions. Nontradizionale will also be expensive. My favorite *non*tradizionale balsamic vinegar is thirty-five dollars for an 8.5-ounce bottle! And that's not even the real stuff! Needless to say, I use it sparingly.

The real *tradizionale* balsamic vinegar is even more expensive than that!

After much tinkering and experimentation, I have come up with a way to make the cheap stuff taste more like the real deal. See the recipe section for my balsamic vinegar.

Dried Figs

The round packages of dried figs from Greece only cost around one dollar. You'll need one package to make the balsamic vinegar.

Virgin Olive Oil

This will set you back anywhere between eight and ten dollars per liter. You'll use olive oil to sauté (not fry) your vegetables and to dress your salads. Virgin olive oil is an integral part of the Mediterranean diet. It lowers oxidized cholesterol, the artery-clogging form of cholesterol.

Rice Cakes

If you can stand to eat them, there are scores of flavors now. These are a far cry from the cardboard versions from a few years ago. In my opinion, they are cardboard nevertheless, whether flavored with cheese or chocolate. Be careful, though. The flavored versions have artificial flavors and chemical preservatives. I would not consider these a health food. There are some new grain cakes out on the market: kamut cakes and spelt cakes. Both spelt and kamut are grains. They may be better for you than rice or wheat because they are higher in protein. You'll find the spelt and kamut rice cakes in health food stores, but not in your local supermarket.

There are also rice cakes with flaxseeds, a great source of omega-3 fatty acids. Like the spelt and kamut rice cakes, these will not be in your local supermarket. You'll need to take a trip to the health food store.

If you have a big appetite, rice cakes are great because they fill you up, especially if you drink a glass of water afterward. When you feel like a crunchy snack, rice cakes fit the bill. For a sweet snack, some jam or honey on a rice cake might satisfy your craving. If you feel like a salty snack, smear some peanut butter on a couple of rice cakes. They are handy to pack as your three o'clock snack.

Frozen Fruits and Vegetables

Although I'm a believer in *fresh* fruits and vegetables, we have to be realistic. You cannot run out to the supermarket every other day to pick up fresh produce. So, stock up on frozen fruits and vegetables. Many frozen fruits and vegetables have higher vitamin contents than fresh ones! This is for a few reasons. First, fresh fruits and vegetables destined for the supermarket are picked before they are ripe. They ship better that way, whereas fruits and vegetables destined for the freezer section are picked when they are ripe. The companies know ripe fruits and vegetables taste better when frozen. If they froze unripe peaches, for example, they would taste like cardboard. So the companies make sure the fruits and vegetables headed for the freezer section are ripe and tasty. Remember, fruits and vegetables contain more vitamins and phytonutrients when ripe. As an added benefit, when fruits and vegetables are frozen, the freezing breaks open the cell walls. Vitamins from inside the cell are released and, thus, available for absorption by your body.

Frozen fruits also taste great, except for frozen strawberries, which do not freeze well. Strawberries develop a spongy consistency and do not have great flavor after they are thawed.

Blueberries, raspberries, blackberries, and cherries freeze very well. Blueberries contain all sorts of phytonutrients and vitamins. An interesting study on blueberries showed that rats that were fed blueberries every day had better memories and better reflexes as they aged.[1] The scientists who performed these experiments were so excited that they started eating blueberries every day as well. See

1. J. A. Joseph and others, "Reversals of Age-Related Declines in Neuronal Signal Transduction, Cognitive, and Motor Behavioral Deficits with Blueberry, Spinach, or Strawberry Dietary Supplementation," *Journal of Neuroscience* 19, no. 18 (1999): 8114–8121.

the recipe for a breakfast blueberry shake, so you too can ward off the effects of aging.

Frozen mangos would be a great choice, but lately, the quality is poor. They taste as if they were not ripe when harvested before freezing. There is an off-brand of mashed mangos from the Dominican Republic. This mango is quite sweet and tasty. Although too stringy to use in a shake, it works well as a topping for yogurt.

Raspberries, mangos, or blackberries are all great on top of yogurt. Take it over the top with granola, wheat germ, and ground flaxseed too. It makes an excellent summer lunch that is full of antioxidants, whole grains, and calcium.

Granola

There are some good supermarket brands of granola. Stay away from anything with HFCS, sugar, or additives you cannot pronounce.

Breakfast Cereals

Pick up one box of sugarless, high-protein cereal as your backup breakfast. Good luck! It will not be easy to find a breakfast cereal fitting the bill. It's best to leave the breakfast cereals to use only in a pinch; they are not a good choice for breakfast, whether it's healthy granola or HFCS-laden Count Chocula. They are all too high in simple carbohydrates (starches and sugars, like high fructose corn syrup) and have virtually no protein. Even adding skim milk will not add enough protein to make it a well-balanced meal. Without protein or fats, after eating a bowl of cereal with skim milk for breakfast, you'll be hungry again in two hours.

Eggs (Not Egg Substitutes)

Egg substitutes are quick and easy—but real eggs are cheaper and certainly better for you since egg substitutes are filled with preservatives and food colorings. Many diets will tell you to avoid egg yolks and to eat only the whites. I personally think there is something healthy in the yolks. For generations, if not for thousands of years, mothers have given their children egg yolks to build strength and improve health. All those generations of moms can't be wrong. It turns out the yolk contains vitamin E, lecithin, B12, and all sorts of essential fatty acids. Many of these fatty acids are delicate and are destroyed in cooking, which is why your grandmother put the *raw* yolk into a drink.

Some studies have shown if you eat eggs in the morning, your hunger is controlled better. I have some big guys in my practice, with big appetites. Instead of a hero sandwich for breakfast, I tell them to have six scrambled eggs, but no bread. Despite their big appetites, they find the eggs really do hold them until it's time for lunch. What's ironic is that those six eggs, scrambled in a pat of butter, probably have fewer calories than the hero sandwich they were accustomed to eating for breakfast.

Try to buy the free-range eggs. They are higher in omega-3 fatty acids.

If you're stuck on the low-fat diet trend (even though low-fat diets don't work, and they are not good for you), you could make an egg white omelet instead of using the egg substitute. Use one egg yolk with four to five egg whites when making your own egg white omelet. The yolk prevents the omelet from sticking to the pan.

A typical Mediterranean meal in our family was a frittata. A frittata is basically a stuffed omelet. My mom would make a frittata as a meal, usually in the summer when it was too hot to cook. She added cheese, leftover sausage or ham, and whatever leftover vegetables she had in the refrigerator. With a salad on the side, a frittata is a quick and easy meal.

Canned Tuna

Buy the canned chunk light tuna in oil. Remember, you want the dark meat tuna called chunk light. The omega-3 fatty acids are higher in chunk light tuna than in albacore. Additionally, the chunk light has less mercury than the solid white or albacore. Don't pour off the oil. Some of the omega-3s and vitamin D end up in the oil. If you're making a salad, use the oil from the can as part of the salad dressing. If you're making a sandwich, don't use mayonnaise. Use the oil in your sandwich and let it soak into the bread, like Europeans do. They chop some celery and onions into the tuna and put a few leaves of lettuce on top. Sometimes a few capers are mixed in with the tuna. Other times, an anchovy or two is laid across the top. Capers and anchovies take the salt content over the top, so go easy with them.

Chicken Broth

Most diet books will tell you to use chicken broth to steam veggies, sauté mushrooms, braise chicken, or make vegetable soup—an endless list of uses. Many of the cheap brands taste awful and are very salty. Some organic brands are pretty good. Beware: the organic brands are expensive. Decide if you have more money or more time. You could save money by making your own chicken broth, especially when chickens are on sale.

If you do decide to make your own chicken broth, do an experiment. Add two tablespoons of vinegar to the water when you start the broth. The acid helps dissolve calcium from the chicken bones. You won't taste the vinegar in the finished broth, and the broth will be enriched with lots of calcium.

Plastic Containers

Save all your plastic containers from the Chinese takeout restaurants. Ask your friends and relatives to save their containers for you. You can buy disposable containers from Ziploc and Glad-Ware at the grocery store, but don't throw them out. Wash them, and reuse them. Scour the church sales for Tupperware containers. You'll need a whole supply because you'll be cooking and saving the leftovers for lunch. You'll be making pots of soup and then freezing them in batches. Don't buy the cheap store brand containers. The lids do not fit well. The container will end up in the garbage after you get frustrated when you try to snap the top onto the container, but spill food on the floor instead.

There is one very important thing to remember about plastic containers. If you use the microwave to reheat food in a plastic container, you must make sure those plastic containers are microwave safe. The plastic containers from the Chinese takeout are *not* microwave safe. Non-microwave-safe containers give off toxic fumes when heated in the microwave. Just to be on the safe side, try not to put any kind of plastic in the microwave ever. Even if it says "microwave safe" on the container, don't do it. It just takes an extra thirty seconds to put the food onto a ceramic plate before sticking it in the microwave.

Organic purists don't store food in plastic ever (or use a microwave for that matter). Olga, the nutritionist at our clinic, stores all her food in glass jars, bowls, or bottles. I use her as a barometer for what is healthy and what is not. If Olga never stores food in plastic, you probably shouldn't either. Start saving the glass jars (tomato sauce, pickles), and in no time, you'll have a whole collection.

However, since glass might not be practical for you, especially if you have a job and a family, there are a few tips to make plastic safer for you. Before you put your cooked food into the plastic container, make sure the food is cool. Never put piping hot food into plastic containers. Think about how nasty water in a plastic bottle tastes after sitting in the sun a couple of hours. Next, never store acidic food in a plastic container. From tomato sauce to lemonade, the acid might leach toxic chemicals from the plastic.

Oatmeal

The slow-cooking variety is best because it has *GLA* (gamma-linolenic acid), an essential fatty acid, which is lost in the quick-cooking varieties. Since it takes almost an hour to cook, make a batch on

Sundays, pack it in four little containers, and have it ready to go. You can spice it up with raisins, brown sugar, and cinnamon.

Cinnamon

Cinnamon is off-the-charts packed with antioxidants. Figure out how and where to use cinnamon. Sprinkle some on sweet potatoes, oatmeal, yogurt, granola, or even in your cup of coffee. Not only is cinnamon high in antioxidants, but also, there is something in cinnamon that *lowers blood sugar levels in diabetics*! This is not some crazy claim by cinnamon farmers in Madagascar. The USDA did extensive research using less than half a teaspoon of cinnamon per day in diabetic patients. They were so excited about the results that they patented the methods they used to process the cinnamon. You can also buy cinnamon capsules, which I absolutely do not recommend. If a little is good, don't assume more is better. It turns out that the good stuff is in the water-soluble part of the cinnamon. The oil-soluble part of the cinnamon can accumulate in your body over time and may be toxic if you overdo it over a long period of time. The USDA patented the process to extract the beneficial water-soluble part of the cinnamon from the oil-soluble part.

Peanut Butter

You can find natural peanut butter at your local supermarket made by Smuckers. Natural peanut butter separates, and you'll see a half-inch of oil on top. You'll need to stir it back together, which is a tedious and messy process. After you mix the oil back into the nut butter, put the jar into the refrigerator. The cold will prevent the oil from separating again. Don't throw out the oil because it contains the essential fatty acids.

You may even be able to find a store with a grinding machine. You can grind your own peanut butter fresh. It's not expensive at $1.99 a pound. If money is not a concern, get some almond butter too. When you get home, put the freshly ground butters in the refrigerator to prevent the oil from separating.

Don't even think about buying reduced-fat peanut butter. The good stuff is in the oils. Do not buy peanut butter if it contains HFCS. You'll need to check the ingredients on the label before you spend your money. If you're accustomed to eating Jiffy or Skippy, you'll notice that natural peanut butter is not as sweet. Good! Now you know what peanut butter is supposed to taste like.

Beans

Beans, beans, beans, in every way, shape, color, and form. Pick up bags of dried beans, lentils, and split peas. If you're on a budget, a bag of dried beans for a dollar goes a long way. See the recipe section for techniques to cook dried beans. It's easier than you think.

If you do not have the time or the desire to cook beans from scratch, keep a stockpile of canned beans in your cabinets. Kidney beans, black beans, or Great Northern beans can all be used in soup or on a salad. You could make your own burritos. Some recipes in this book will call for cannellini beans; pick up a few cans of these smooth and delicate-tasting white beans.

Cans of baked beans or Boston-baked beans don't fall into this category. They are a processed food, with artificial coloring and trans fats. If you love baked beans, you'll need to make your own.

Brown Rice

Expand your horizons with brown rice. Try other grains such as quinoa or couscous. Try some of the varieties of wild rice from the supermarket for a change of pace. If you live in an area with an Indian or Pakistani neighborhood, take a trip to one of their food stores. On lower Lexington Avenue in Manhattan, there are several Indian shops and restaurants. The whole area is filled with the scents of Indian spices. Chefs from all over the country go there to shop for spices and browse the shelves. These stores have more varieties of wild rice, black rice, and red rice than you ever knew existed. The same goes for the lentils—red lentils, yellow lentils, black lentils. The prices cannot be beat either.

Notice *white* rice is not on this list. You may hate brown rice. Okay, you can eat white rice, but only in moderation. No more than one ice cream scoop of rice at a meal.

Barley

A bag of barley is exceedingly inexpensive. You can use it in soups or as a side dish with chicken or stewed meat.

Pasta

Don't buy a lot of pasta. A couple of boxes will do. You'll be eating pasta in moderation only. One cup is the serving size for pasta. Try to buy whole wheat pasta if you can stand the taste. The new versions are so much better than they were a few years ago. The imported Italian varieties of whole wheat pasta are really good but very expensive. If you don't like whole wheat pasta, try semolina pasta. Don't skimp on the pasta, even if the cheaper brands are on sale. You won't be eating much of it, so you can afford to spend a bit more. De Cecco is an excellent brand and is readily available in most supermarkets. De Cecco whole wheat pasta is also quite tasty, a vast improvement over the cardboard version of whole wheat pasta from twenty years ago. Experiment. Have fun while trying new foods.

Tomato Sauce

Here you'll need to invest some money. The cheaper sauces that are two jars for three dollars contain HCFS, additives, preservatives, and artificial ingredients. The more expensive brands don't have HFCS but are twice as expensive, at three dollars for one jar. You might even consider making your own pasta sauce. It's time consuming, though. If you work, have kids, and a spouse/partner who needs attention, go ahead and buy prepared sauces. Your precious time is better spent preparing salads and vegetables.

Canned Plum Tomatoes

You won't need many cans, thankfully (the cans are really very heavy to carry home from the supermarket). You'll need a can or two for a few of the bean and lentil recipes. You'll need a few more if you intend to make your own tomato sauce for pasta. The best plum tomatoes are from San Marzano in Italy, near Naples. There is something about San Marzano. It might be the volcanic soil, the blazing sunshine, or the sea breezes. These tomatoes are especially sweet and bright red.

Chicken Breasts

Chicken cutlets or chicken fingers are a perfect snack when eaten with a piece of fruit. Try different sauces: barbecue sauce, Thai peanut sauce, tandoori sauce, or hoisin sauce, my personal favorite. Once or twice a week, make a pile of chicken fingers. You could even make two piles in two different flavors. A piece of chicken plus a piece of fruit is an especially perfect snack for diabetics, who need a bit of protein, fat, and carbohydrates to maintain their blood sugar at a constant level in between meals. A piece of fruit with a piece of chicken is also a good snack for the people who have a long commute home or work twelve-hour shifts. They need a substantial snack to get them through the long afternoon until dinnertime.

Brown Sugar

Brown sugar is regular white sugar with some of the molasses added back. It's better for you than regular sugar because molasses has minerals, antioxidants, and is high in calcium. Brown sugar will be used in your oatmeal and for sprinkling on top of butternut or acorn squash. Remember that sugar, whether it's brown, white, tan, or black (like in molasses), is sugar nevertheless. Go easy!

Pine Nuts, Walnuts, Pecans, Almonds

Nuts can be sprinkled on a salad or used as a garnish on sautéed vegetables. A little goes a long way; you cannot possibly use up a whole package in ten or twelve weeks. They'd go rancid by then. You can keep nuts fresh by storing them in the freezer.

Make little snack packs of nuts and dried fruit to pack in your purse or in the glove compartment. Never get caught starving on the subway or in the car.

Emergency Foods

Emergency foods are the quick, healthy snacks you want to keep in your purse or glove compartment for those times when you're stuck on the highway or on the subway. These are great if you're running out of the house and realize you're a little hungry. If you like bars, Zone Bars are great. They have protein, carbohydrates, and fats in just the right proportion. For those of you without a sweet tooth, bars may not be to your liking. Small bags of nuts are also great, especially walnuts, which are high in omega-3s. Trail mix, dried fruit, or even bananas make a perfect portable, healthy snack. Remember, these are only snacks. We are not talking about a full three-course meal to bring as your three o'clock snack.

Buy Your Perishables and Food for the Week

Perishables are your fruits and vegetables for the week, assuming you only go to the market once a week. If you are in the habit of stopping into the greengrocer every couple of days, you can spread out your shopping over the week.

Garlic, Onion, Carrots, Celery

Chopped and sautéed together, garlic, onion, carrots, and celery are the basis and flavoring for soups, bean dishes, and sautéed veg-etables. In France, the mixture of onion, carrot, and celery is called *mirepoix*. In Hispanic cooking, the mixture consists of garlic, pep-per, and cilantro, and is called *sofrito*. You'll find something similar in almost every cuisine of the world.

If you like raw carrots as a snack, try to find carrots with the tops still on. They will be more expensive, but buy them once just to taste the difference. They are moist and have a much sweeter flavor. You may never go back to those old, dried-out orange torpedoes they sell in plastic bags. If you do buy the carrots with the leafy tops, cut off the tops when you get home from the supermarket. If you leave the green leaves on, nutrients are drawn from the root into the leaves, and the carrots will lose some of their flavor and sweetness.

Lemons

Squeeze lemon juice on your salad instead of vinegar. The French and the Italians do this on their tuna salads. Splash some lemon juice on sautéed vegetables, but don't add the juice too soon. The juice can become bitter with cooking, so splash it on toward the end of the cooking process.

Before you squeeze a lemon, roll it under the heel of your hand with pressure. The pressure helps to break down the fibers, so more juice can be squeezed from each lemon. You could pop the lemons in the microwave for ten seconds for the same effect. Health food purists don't microwave anything, but you can squeeze your lemon whichever way you prefer.

Milk

Skim, low-fat, or regular milk—the choice is yours. Some people refuse to buy low-fat milk because they don't like the taste. Others are stuck on the low-fat trend. If you do use whole milk, remember calories count. Whole milk has more calories than skim or 2 percent milk. On the other hand, skim milk doesn't control your hunger as well. There is no right or wrong answer. I will not argue about politics, religion, or the fat content of milk. Buy the milk you like.

Yogurt

Don't buy sweetened yogurt. Don't buy the nonfat variety. Don't buy yogurt with artificial sweeteners. They all taste like plastic soup.

Buy as close to natural as you can get. Some of the organic brands you can find in your supermarket, like Stonyfield Farm, are good. If you can find Greek-style yogurt, go for it. For a long time, there was only one brand of Greek-style yogurt I could ever find: Fage. Since people are now discovering delicious Greek-style yogurt, there are more brands available. Try one of these brands of Greek-style yogurt just once. It's thicker and richer. One taste will take you on a trip to the Greek island of Mykonos without ever leaving your kitchen. This thick, rich, and creamy yogurt is so much more satisfying than watery American-style yogurt. Greek-style yogurt is a bit more expensive and is higher in calories, but you will eat less of it because it's so much more filling.

When there is some fat in food, the flavors are sensed by the taste buds better. The fat is a vehicle to transport the taste from the food to your palate. That's what this rich Greek yogurt does. You can taste the yogurt, and you need less of it to be satisfied.

Salad Greens

You'll be eating a salad every day, if not twice a day. Mix it up: arugula, butter lettuce, mesclun greens, romaine—whatever looks fresh at the supermarket. Since I hate the task of washing salad greens, I recommend buying the packaged romaine lettuce. It's always fairly clean and easy to chop up into a salad. Endive and radicchio are also easy to use but expensive. Either way, you still need to give the greens at least one washing. Even the prewashed salad greens need another rinse before you eat them. Until the outbreaks of E. coli from contaminated spinach, I never bothered to wash the prewashed salads a second time. Now I always do. E. coli are bacteria from the feces of cows. Vegetables grown near cow pastures can be contaminated as rainwater washes the cow manure downstream.

Fruits and Vegetables

See what fruit and vegetables look good at the market. Depending on the season, oranges, grapes, and apples are always a good choice. Grapes are vital to the Mediterranean diet. Eat grapes every day when they are in season. Forget the peaches, nectarines, and melons unless they smell like a peach, nectarine, or melon. Remember, they are unripe when picked, so they can be shipped long distances. Fruits picked before ripening never develop their full, complex flavors, even if you sit the fruit on the windowsill to ripen.

Become creative with the vegetables: collard greens, Swiss chard, broccoli rabe, cauliflower, and asparagus—get whatever looks good. Go with the seasons: greens in the springtime and winter squash in the autumn. Get wild: try something you've never tried before, like fennel, celery root (celeriac), or dandelion.

Potatoes, Yams, Sweet Potatoes

Go easy with the starches. You can have a potato every day, but then you'll need to cut down on your starches in other meals. If possible, stick to sweet potatoes and yams. Their beautiful orange color tells you they have higher carotene content than white potatoes. Diabetics and prediabetics are under the mistaken impression that they cannot eat sweet potatoes. The body absorbs sugars in sweet potatoes and yams slowly, so they are safe for diabetics to eat. Still, eat them in moderation only, and you absolutely cannot put sugar and marshmallows on top. Who invented that recipe? Yams and sweet potatoes are healthy and nutritious. Adding sugar and marshmallows turns them into an artery-clogging, mind-numbing, sugar-blast.

Kosher Salt

You need to buy a box of kosher salt, which is large-grain salt. You'll recognize the big blue box when you see it. This is the salt to cook with. You'll see the difference. A little bit of kosher salt goes a long way. You'll use less salt in the long run.

Spices and Herbs

You don't need a lot of spices or herbs to start. Black pepper and parsley will do. If you intend to make beans, buy a one-dollar bag of bay leaves in either the spice section or the ethnic section of the supermarket. Make sure you have a box of coarse kosher salt, and you're all set.

Most vegetables, if you buy them fresh, do not need a lot of spices to mask the taste. Fifty percent of the time, the vegetables I cook are only seasoned with salt, pepper, and garlic. Other times, a splash of lemon juice on asparagus or mint on artichokes adds an interesting twist. This is the Italian way of cooking vegetables. Buy the freshest possible ingredients, and let their flavor shine through.

After you buy salt, pepper, parsley, and bay leaves, you'll not need much else for a while. Wait to spend money on herbs and spices until you understand your cooking style and how often you'll be cooking. Later, you can add basil, sage, thyme, and rosemary to your grocery list. Fresh herbs are always better. If you have the time and the inclination, wash a batch of fresh herbs. Let the leaves dry off (but not dry out), and then freeze them in plastic bags. That way, you'll always have a supply of "fresh" herbs on hand. Washing and drying your own herbs may be far too time-consuming for you. Go ahead. Use the dried herbs. You have better ways to spend your precious time.

Secondary Things to Buy When You Have Some Extra Money

These are items you may not have tried yet, so don't buy too much.

Capers

If you can find capers preserved in salt, go for them. These dried, salted capers are sold in ethnic Italian neighborhoods. They are not expensive at all. Chances are you won't find dry, salt-packed capers in your local supermarket. The jars of capers packed in salted water are just fine. Use capers for chicken and fish dishes. Capers last forever in the refrigerator. Most recipes only call for one or two tablespoons, so a small jar will last you a long time. If you do buy the dried, salted capers, they need to be soaked in water for a few minutes and rinsed before cooking.

Capers are another one of those foods with a spectacular amount of antioxidants.

Anchovies

Don't say yuck until you've tried them; anchovies are great on a salad. *Anchovies on salad!* You might think that's disgusting, but real Caesar salad is made with anchovies. A few anchovies blended with garlic, olive oil, and vinegar is a tasty salad dressing.

If you take a trip to France or Italy, you might find an anchovy or two on top of your tuna sandwich. Instead of mayonnaise, your tuna sandwich would be sprinkled with olive oil and vinegar, or olive oil and lemon juice. Delizioso!

Sardines

On the supermarket shelf, right next to the anchovies, are the sardines. Pick up a can, just one can, to try it out. You might want to try the boneless, skinless sardines first. Sardines are full of vitamin D, vitamin A, and omega-3 fatty acids. Put sardines on a salad. Eat them on crackers for a snack like they do in Spain.

If you can stand it, get the sardines with the bones still in. If you eat the thin, crunchy bones, you'll get an excellent and easily absorbable blast of calcium. My sister loves sardines this way, though it's a bit much, even for me.

Sardines are actually very, very good for you. There is even a book called *The Sardine Diet*. Imagine that! Someone wrote a diet book about sardines.

Flaxseed Oil

Flaxseed oil is expensive, and you must only purchase organic brands of flaxseed oil. You won't be using much of the oil, so a small bottle will last you several weeks. Actually, a small bottle will last a few months. You must keep this oil in the refrigerator, and you can *never, never* cook with flaxseed oil. You can use a table-spoon in your salad dressing on the days you're not eating seafood or walnuts. You may pour a tablespoon into you breakfast shake. Better yet…

Cod-Liver Oil

Generations of grandmothers have been giving cod-liver oil to their children and grandchildren. Read the chapter on vitamin D for more information about the benefits of cod-liver oil.

Avoid Like the Plague

Trans fats or any foods made with trans fats:

> This includes Crisco. Avoid Crisco and other vegetable shortenings. On the rare occasions you need to fry something, use lard or canola oil. On the even rarer occasions you want to make a piecrust, use butter or lard.

High fructose corn syrup or any foods made with it

Frankenfoods or any food made with ingredients you cannot pronounce:

> We get enough chemicals from mercury in our fish, hormones in our cattle, pesticides on our vegetables, and smog in our air. We don't have to help the process along with these fake foods.

Fat-free cheese

Fat-free sour cream

Fat-free, sugar-free yogurt

Fat-free yogurt, or frozen yogurt, with high sugar content

Fat-free cookies and cakes with high sugar content

Margarine, even those margarines made from healthy oil and claim to help reduce your cholesterol

Cooking sprays:

> You're better off using a small amount of oil in the

bottom of your baking pans. The cooking sprays turn into a hard and sticky substance after baking, which makes it impossible to scrub your pans clean.

Soda (diet or regular):

The carbonation in soda binds to calcium in the intestines and makes it unavailable for absorption by the body. If decreasing calcium absorption weren't bad enough, soda (especially colas) may actually leach calcium from your bones, contributing to osteoporosis. People with osteoporosis also lose bone density in their jaw, so teeth become loose. To add insult to injury, the acids in soda then rot your teeth. Why does anyone spend money on this stuff? Carbonated mineral waters, like San Pelegrino or Perrier, are acceptable and are, quite possibly, a good source of trace minerals.

Processed luncheon meats:

These are full of chemicals and may even increase your risk of colon cancer! There is a new term you'll be hearing on the news soon: advanced glycation end-products. These chemicals are abbreviated as AGE and are produced when foods are cooked at high temperatures. AGEs form between sugars and proteins. They are the tasty, crisp, brown crust on a grilled steak. AGEs are bad for you, especially if you are a diabetic. Luncheon meats are very high in AGEs. Stay away from them. Diet soda is also high in AGEs. Who would have ever guessed! That's another good reason to avoid soda.

Soymilk:

If you're gung ho about eating healthy, do not buy soymilk and assume you're doing your body a favor. Many health food purists would caution you against eating soy-based foods, unless the soy has been fermented, like tofu or tempeh. It's especially important to avoid soy-based foods if you're having problems with fertility.

If you have been trying to become pregnant without success, avoid soymilk and even tofu and tempeh. Soy has phytoestrogens, which are hormones from plant sources. They are close enough to human estrogens that they actually do cross over and have hormone effects in humans. That's why women use soy to relieve the symptoms of menopause, even though it has never been proven to work. Soy is also believed to decrease a woman's chances of getting breast cancer; although, once again, it has never been proven. In Japan, where they eat soy every day, the rate of breast cancer is quite low. The flip side of the coin is that Japan has a low birthrate. Scientists think the lower rate of fertility is related to their high intake of soy. Realistically, it would take an awful lot of soy to affect your fertility, but if you are having trouble becoming pregnant, just avoid soy. And at the same time, watch your starch and sugar intake. Diabetes, prediabetes, and polycystic ovary syndrome all result in reduced fertility. High intake of starches and sugars put you at high risk for these three diseases. All three are the same disease really. Each one is just at a different point along the spectrum of impaired glucose metabolism.

Chapter Fifteen

Use Some Common Sense

I
t would make sense to spread your food out among the three big categories of foods: carbohydrates, protein, and fats. However, we are all hooked on eating foods made out of seeds or roots. Think about the things you eat the most: rice (a seed), potatoes (a root), bread and pasta (wheat is a seed), and soda (the HFCS is from corn, which is a seed). Since the seed or the root is where the new plant grows from, it's packed with calories, so the new plant can grow. Some patients tell me that peas are the only green vegetable they will eat. This is not a surprise, since peas are a starchy vegetable.

One patient swore she only ate 1,500 calories per day. She couldn't understand why she was so heavy, why her body fat percentage was very high, why she was not losing weight, and why she had no energy. She was really quite obese and had a disease called *sleep apnea*. Every night, she needed to wear a face mask attached to a machine to help her breath. If she lost weight, it might have improved her sleep apnea. Then, she would not have needed to wear the mask every night. It's no fun to sleep with a mask on your face.

When we reviewed her food intake, she ate the same thing every day: a plain bagel for breakfast without butter or jam, a bag of pretzels for lunch, and a big bowl of pasta for dinner. She was absolutely correct. It was a very low-fat diet. When we counted up the calories, she was right again. She only ate 1,500 calories each day. Yet without any vegetables or protein, it was no wonder she felt tired all the time, was constipated, and could not lose weight.

Another one of my patients has a particular form of diabetes as a result of his HIV medications. His arms and legs are super-skinny, and his abdomen (belly) is huge. I hate to insult a patient, but he really does look pregnant. He needs to cut out all the starches and sweets in his diet and concentrate on eating protein, healthy fats, and vegetables. We have been going through the list of starches to avoid over and over. Just like they are always cleverly finding something else sweet to drink, my diabetic patients crave starches. I told him to eliminate pasta, bread, and rice from his diet. Well, he did that. He ate yucca, potatoes, plantains, bananas, and other starchy root vegetables or fruits instead. Learn from his mistake. Subtract the starchy vegetables, and replace them with vegetables like spinach, salad greens, peppers, zucchini, cauli-flower, broccoli, and so on.

Sometimes I ask a patient who is especially starch-addicted to do an experiment for one week. Just for one week, no starches. In order to do this, someone would also need to increase the healthy fats in their diet for the week. Without the extra healthy fats, someone cutting out all starches would be hungry all the time. Somehow, somewhere between my lips and the patient's ears, something gets lost in the translation. One patient was going to do the experiment for a week. She is overweight and diabetic, but she has a great outlook on life. She loves avocados, so she was really happy to do the experiment. She came back after a week. She told me how much she loved being able to eat an avocado every day. Her weight didn't change, her blood sugars were the same, and she looked and felt the same. How come? Well, she added the avocado but never stopped eating big bowls of pasta, rice, and potatoes. She looked surprised. "I can't eat pasta during the experiment?" No, you cannot eat pasta or rice or bread during the experiment. "Can I eat waffles or muffins?" No waffles. No muffins. "Does that mean I can't eat pancakes?" Pancakes!

Avoid Simple Carbohydrates: Starches and Sweets

It's obvious from their stories that these three patients are carbo-hydrate addicts. The first common sense rule is to avoid simple carbohydrates. Carbohydrates are used by the body for energy. Muscle is not made from carbohydrates, nor can carbohydrates be used to make hormones or build cell walls. Hormones and cell walls are examples of substances and structures in the body made out of fats. Carbohydrates can only be used for energy, or if eaten in excess, stored as fat. *Complex* carbohydrates include all your fruits, vegetables, and whole grains like brown rice. Even legumes (lentils, peanuts, etc.) and beans should be considered complex carbohydrates. Although beans and legumes contain a small amount of protein, they are mostly made of carbohydrates. *Simple* carbohydrates include starches such as white rice, white potatoes, and pasta, as well as table sugar and high fructose corn syrup. Fruit juice should be considered a simple carbohydrate, which is why you need to limit juices. Juices you can see through, like apple juice, are really not on the program. You'll end up like our friend, the Mack truck, if you drink apple juice all day. Cran-berry juice is another see-through juice to limit. It's sweetened with loads of sugar. Eat lots of vegetables and fruits, and avoid the starches and sugars.

Sugars and starches are converted into glucose by the body very rapidly. The glucose load causes the pancreas to pump out insulin. The insulin causes fat cells to take up the glucose and con-vert it to fat. The *simple* sugars cause more of an insulin response than the *complex* carbohydrates. How fast this occurs is called a food's *glycemic index.*

The glycemic index of a food is a measure of how fast that food is turned into glucose by the body. Something like Wonder Bread is turned into sugar almost immediately. It has a glycemic index of one hundred. Foods like vegetables, nuts, beans, and fruits, have lower gylcemic indexes, of twenty or thirty or forty. It takes the body longer to turn them into sugar. You do not want to eat a high-glycemic-index diet. A good example of a high-glycemic-index diet is what our 1,500-calorie friend ate every day: a bagel for breakfast, pretzels for lunch, and pasta for dinner. This is a setup for diabetes. First of all, every meal needs to be well balanced: protein, fats, and carbohydrates. Secondly, get rid of the simple carbohydrates, like table sugar, high fructose corn syrup, white bread, pasta, and white rice. You're much better off eating complex carbohydrates, such as whole grains, fruits, and vegetables, instead of the refined grain products. The simple sugars and refined carbohydrates not only make the body pump out insulin, but their calories are *empty calories*, which means the vitamins and minerals were removed during processing. These processed foods provide you with calories, but not with nutrients.

Foods with a high glycemic index are especially unhealthy for people with diabetes or prediabetes. Calorie for calorie, people with diabetes or prediabetes lose *less* weight if they eat a high-glycemic-index diet.[1] Yes, let's say you have diabetes, as does your next-door neighbor. You both start a diet eating 1,500 calories every day. If you eat vegetables, beans, lentils, fruit, meat, and fish, but your neighbor eats bagels, pretzels, and pasta, you'll lose more weight, even though you're both eating the same number of calories each day!

Here is a chart of the glycemic indexes of a few foods. By all means, this is not a complete list.

1. C. B. Ebbeling and others, "Effects of a Low-Glycemic Load vs Low-Fat Diet in Obese Young Adults: A Randomized Trial," *Journal of the American Medical Association* 297 (2007): 2092–2102.

HIGH	MEDIUM HIGH	MEDIUM	LOW (GOOD)
White Bread	Carrot	Pasta	Nuts
Instant Rice	Banana	Orange	Oatmeal (slow cooked)
Corn Flakes	Corn	Peas	Apple
Instant Potatoes	Raisins	Beans	Pear
Puffed Wheat	Apricot	Milk	Cherries
Puffed Rice	Mango	Yogurt	Barley

You can see a trend in the chart. Processed foods have high gylcemic indexes. Sweet fruits and starchy vegetables have medium-high glycemic indexes. Complex foods have low glycemic indexes. You really don't have to worry about the specifics. If you stay away from processed foods, you'll be avoiding all the high-gly-cemic-index foods. Michael Pollan, a famous journalist who writes about food issues, says that eating processed foods is like "main-lining sugar."[2] We are bringing up a whole generation of children addicted to sugar! I read an interesting article about Applebee's restaurants. The director of public relations said that they have needed to change the dessert recipes through the years; they can't make desserts sweet enough for their customers.[3] America has become a country of sugar addicts.

When planning your diet, minimize the pasta, rice, corn, and potatoes. It's so easy to eat a big bowl of rice or pasta at dinner. Those starches will really pack on the pounds. Every single one of my obese patients is crazy about starches, be it pasta, potatoes, rice, or bread. If you do eat rice or pasta, choose brown rice over white rice, or if you can stand to eat it, whole wheat pasta instead

2. Michael Pollan, "Unhappy Meals," *New York Times*, January 28, 2008.
3. Kim Severson, "A Craving for Riblets and Change at Applebee's," *New York Times*, August 19, 2008.

of white pasta. Whole wheat products still have the bran and the germ. These are the parts that contain the vitamins, minerals, and antioxidants. There is a lot of data now suggesting that two servings a day of *whole* grains, like oatmeal, barley, bulgur (whole wheat), or wild rice, help prevent diabetes.

More importantly, if you count calories, you're only allowed 200 calories of starch on this diet. That's right! Only a cup of pasta, half a bagel, or two-thirds cup of brown rice—for the whole day! The rest of your carbohydrates will be coming from the truly complex carbohydrates. Unrefined, in their natural state, sweet potatoes, beans, grains, lentils, vegetables, and fruits will be the source of your complex carbohydrates. This is common sense. It's not rocket science. Look around. Your friends and relatives, the ones who eat potatoes, rice, and pasta for breakfast, lunch, and dinner, all washed down with soda, are slow and sluggish. Your friends and relatives, the ones who love their salads, vegetables, and fruits, but limit the bread, rice, and pasta, are healthy and full of energy.

Don't get me wrong. You need carbohydrates in your diet. Have you ever wondered why you lost weight on a low-carbohydrate diet, like Atkins, but then gained it all back? Your body was sending you a message that something was missing. The fiber from fruits and vegetables keeps your colon moving. The vitamins, minerals, and phytochemicals from fruits and vegetables help your cells heal themselves and protect themselves from the effects of free radicals. Your body was screaming for the vitamins, minerals, and phytochemicals found in fruits and vegetables. You simply could not keep eating an Atkins-type diet for more than a few days. Atkins is really a very good diet, if you do it right. Most people don't; they cheat by eating bread, pasta, and potatoes, when they are only allowed a salad. Just as people cannot resist the urge to scratch an itch, they cannot resist the urge to eat starchy carbohydrates. The point is you must change your eating habits into a healthy pattern you can maintain for life. Something you'll be happy with for the next ten, twenty, or fifty years. You need a diet and a lifestyle that will keep you healthy, happy, and satisfied for the rest of your life.

Reduce Your Fat Intake

The next common sense rule is to reduce your fat intake. "Reduce my fat intake?" you must be wondering. "Didn't the last one hundred pages tell me to eat more fats? Which one is it?" This one, I'm afraid, we're going to have to play by ear and use common sense. Fats are important for health, but ounce for ounce, fat has twice the calories of carbohydrates. One ounce of a high-fat food like cheese contains 100 calories, whereas one ounce of protein, like a grilled skinless chicken breast, contains 50 calories. Since about 30 percent of your daily calories should come from fat, you'll need to figure out your healthy level of fat intake, one that does not cause weight gain. We could get scientific about it. You could weigh every piece of food and calculate your fat calories for the day. Divide your fat calories by your total calories to calculate your percent fat intake for the day. You'd be able to ensure that exactly 30 percent of your calories come from fats every single day, but you wouldn't have much time for anything else.

In my practice, I see people falling into two extremes. Either people add too much fat back to their diet, or too little. Too much fat will add too many calories, and you won't lose weight. Too little fat in your diet and you'll be hungry and unhealthy. As a matter of fact, some people limit the fats so much that it actually prevents them from losing weight. One of my patients is a husky Mexican guy. He's a construction worker, so he does plenty of "exercise" at work. As if that isn't enough activity, when he gets home from work, he grabs his two sons and takes them to the park to play soccer. But he never lost a pound on his diet. He was eating a very low-fat diet, and he limited his starches. For breakfast, his wife would make him egg white omelets. She would eat the extra yolks instead of throwing them out. She is thin, so that should have been a hint right there. For lunch, he would have tuna packed in water on whole wheat bread and a piece of fruit. At dinner, he would eat grilled chicken without the skin and a salad without dressing. Still, he never lost a pound. I told him to add fats back into his diet. Eat the egg yolks. Put olive oil on your salad. Use tuna packed in olive oil. Well, wasn't he surprised when he lost fourteen pounds in three months by eating more fats! More fats meant more calories, but he still lost weight. Fats are important for every aspect of health, including weight loss.

Go back to the fat chapters and read them again. Remember, certain fats are better than others. For instance, olive oil may actually protect you against heart attacks. The oils in certain nuts, like walnuts, may help the immune system and prevent heart attacks. For your health, you need to *eliminate* all the bad fats and add good fats to your diet. To lose weight, you need to *limit* high-fat foods like cheese, nuts, and oils. Yes, nuts and olive oil are good for you, but if you eat a pound of nuts every day, you'll gain weight. Remember, everything in moderation. Add a *small* amount of olive oil to your salads, not a cup. Eat a handful or two of nuts, not a pound, every day.

Make Every Meal Well Balanced

Each meal should be well balanced, meaning each meal (and every snack if you can) should contain some protein, carbohydrates, and fat.

Let me explain in greater detail. If you need 1,600 calories every day to be healthy, about 30 percent, more or less, of those calories should come from fat. You could push it and go for a lower-fat diet, getting, let's say, 20 percent of your calories from fat. You cannot be compulsive about it. Some days you'll eat more fats. Other days, for example in the summer when you're eating more salads and fruits, less of your calories will be from fats. Just aim for anything in the range of 20 to 40 percent of your calories from fats. A diet with less than 20 percent fat is simply not good for you and is a very difficult diet to maintain.

Another 30 percent, more or less, of your calories should come from protein. We get plenty of protein in our American diet. You do not have to worry about increasing your protein intake. I have never seen a case of protein-calorie malnutrition in East Harlem. It's much more likely you'll need to reduce your protein intake and shift to eating more complex carbohydrates. The exceptions to this are the people, like our 1,500-calorie friend, eating bagels, pretzels, and pasta. She was eating no protein at all. She needed to add fish, chicken, and meat to her diet, pronto!

The next 40 to 50 percent of your calories will be from carbohydrates. Let me digress for a moment. There are some high-carbohydrate diets out there, like Ornish and Pritikin. These are very difficult diets to stay on for the long haul. On Pritikin, for example, 10 percent of your calories would be from fats, 10 percent from protein, and 80 percent from complex carbohydrates. There is some scientific evidence showing a lower risk of heart disease in those who eat a diet high in fiber and complex carbohydrates. But don't fool yourself. Eating pasta, bread, potatoes, and rice all day does not qualify as Pritikin. Those diets, like the Pritikin, focus on the truly complex carbohydrates: fruits, vegetables, beans, and legumes. There are no refined starches or sugars on Pritikin. Eating a bagel for breakfast, pretzels for lunch, and pasta for dinner does *not* qualify as Pritikin.

So let's go back to the issue at hand. About half of your calories should come from complex carbohydrates, like vegetables, whole grains, beans, lentils, and nuts. The reality is you aren't going to be weighing your food and calculating percentages of fats, carbohydrates, and protein. Here is a simpler way to estimate proportions.

If you divide your plate into three sections, one will be for your meat, one for your vegetable, and one for your starch. Keep the starches as close to nature as possible. Your starch should be a baked potato instead of bread, wild rice instead of white rice. The section of the plate with your starch should be one-third or smaller. Don't try to fudge it and have the starch take up half the plate. If anything, have your salad and vegetables take up half the plate, and the starch and meat take up a quarter each.

Then, you know the little dish on the side? That's the plate you used to use as a dessert plate. It's your salad plate now. Eat a salad every day. If you're eating cabbage soup for dinner, you can skip the salad. If your vegetable is a pile of sautéed spinach, you can skip the salad. On days you're not having a salad, put fruit on the little plate for dessert. There are other exceptions to the one-third rule. There will be days when dinner is simply a bowl of split pea soup, lentil soup, or minestrone. A bowl of a hardy soup is satisfying as a meal, but it might be low in protein for you. If you become hungry two hours after eating a bowl of soup for dinner, it means the soup did not have enough protein or fat or both in it.

If you divide your plate into three sections for the meat, starch, and vegetable, and include the dessert plate for a salad or fruit, you might ask "Where is the section for my fat allotment?" The fat takes care of itself. If you are putting oil on your salad, eating some meat, and sautéing your vegetables in olive oil, you have met your fat allotment for that meal.

As you can see, this is not the kind of diet that tells you exactly what to eat for breakfast, lunch, and dinner. You need to make those decisions for yourself. This is not the kind of diet that promises you a twenty-pound weight loss in two weeks. That's an unrealistic goal, and one that you would not be able to maintain. The information given here are broad brushstrokes for a diet that will keep you healthy. Use some common sense, and make every meal well balanced with some protein, complex carbohydrates, and healthy fats.

Chapter Sixteen

Multivitamins, Calcium, and Other Supplements

I
f you're on a diet but are otherwise pretty healthy, a multivitamin might be a good idea, though not really necessary if you're eating lots of fruits and vegetables. A multivitamin is especially unnecessary if you're using one of those powdered green extracts (mentioned in chapter 12) in your morning shake. A scoop of one of these extracts has the equivalent of five servings of fruits and vegetables. If you have diabetes, a multivitamin is a good idea because you need plenty of antioxidants. Diabetics make free radicals faster than the government prints new money, so you need more antioxidants to combat them.

If you do decide to take a multivitamin, be sure to choose a high-quality one. No surprise here: it will be expensive. So how you do tell a good multivitamin from a bad one? Don't go by the price. I would not recommend some more expensive ones. You'll be able to tell a good one from a bad one by looking at the vitamin E content and the beta-carotene content. (Beta-carotene may be listed as β-carotene.)

The vitamin E content should be listed as *mixed* tocopherols. Vitamin E comes in a variety of configurations: alpha, beta, delta, and gamma. You want a mixture of these configurations. The same rule applies for carotene. If the multivitamin has beta-carotene alone, don't buy it. It should contain *mixed* carotenoids. Although beta-carotene is the best known of the carotenes, there are actually hundreds of varieties, called carotenoids, with names like lycopene, phytofluene, lutein, and zeaxanthin. Carotenoids are important for health. For example, lutein, found in tomatoes, and zeaxanthin, found in spinach and kale, reduce the risk of becoming blind from age-related macular degeneration.

When you're looking for a multivitamin containing mixed tocopherols and mixed carotenoids, the label might look like this:

Vitamin A (natural mixed carotenoids, including beta-carotene, alpha-carotene, lutein, zeaxanthin)	10,000 IU	200%
Vitamin C	2,000 mg	3,330%
Vitamin D3 (cholecalciferol)	2,000 IU	500%
Natural Vitamin E (d-alpha tocopheryl succinate and high gamma mixed tocopherols)	800 IU	660%

From this label, you can see the vitamin E has mixed tocopherols as well as a mixture of carotenoids. Mixed carotenoids are especially important. In a Finnish study, middle-aged male smokers were given a beta-carotene supplement.[1] Since people with higher levels of beta-carotene in their blood are less likely to develop cancer, scientists figured, "Hey! Let's give some people who are at a really high risk of cancer some beta-carotene. Maybe

---

1. O. P. Heinonen and D. Albanes, "The Effect of Vitamin E and Beta-Carotene on the Incidence of Lung Cancer and Other Cancers in Male Smokers," *New England Journal of Medicine* 330, no. 15 (1994): 1029–1035.

the beta-carotene will prevent cancer in some of them." Who do you think is at a really high risk of cancer? That's right, smokers! The researchers were hoping they could prevent lung cancer from developing in some of the men.

However, the study was terminated *early* because the men who took the beta-carotene supplement developed cancer *more* often! How could this be? Vitamins are supposed to be good for you!

Well, scientists have been trying to come up with an explanation. First of all, people with the highest levels of carotenes in their blood are people who are eating lots of fruits and vegetables in the first place. This is where natural beta-carotene comes from—fruits and vegetables—not from one of those chemical factories along the New Jersey Turnpike.

A high level of beta-carotene in someone's blood is a "marker" for a healthy lifestyle. These are the people who make it a point to eat a lot of fruits and vegetables. People who eat lots of fruits and vegetables are more likely to exercise regularly. Those who exercise regularly are less likely to smoke. So the high level of beta-carotene is a "marker" for someone who eats healthy, exercises, doesn't smoke, and thus, is less likely to develop lung cancer. A couch potato cannot make up for a lifetime of cheeseburgers and cigarettes by taking a vitamin for three to six months; however, this does not explain why taking the supplement made the smokers more likely to develop cancer.

One explanation for the apparent contradiction of a beta-carotene supplement resulting in more cancer is that there are hundreds of carotenoids. Beta-carotene is not as good an antioxidant as the others. By taking a beta-carotene supplement, it overwhelms the carotene receptors in the intestine and does not allow the absorption of other carotenoids that are better antioxidants. Yet, that does not make much sense to me. My favorite explanation, one that does make sense, is that, when you take megadoses of antioxidants in a pill form, it actually has the opposite effect. They become toxic. The antioxidants turn into an oxidant and damage the delicate machinery inside your cells. A little bit of perfume is intoxicatingly beautiful. Too much and you'll give yourself an asthma attack.

Beta-carotene is just another example of how you cannot take the magic ingredient out of a food, put it in a pill, and expect miracles. Until this question is resolved, it's best to use food as your source of carotenoids, or a supplement containing mixed carotenoids. The carotenoids are precursors of vitamin A; they are converted by the body into vitamin A. It's impossible to overdose on carotenoids but very possible to overdose on vitamin A, especially if it's synthetic and you take high doses over a long period of time. There is a long list of symptoms of vitamin A toxicity, including dry skin, hair loss, irritability, loss of appetite, and insomnia. Thus, you should avoid multivitamins that have vitamin A instead of carotenoids. Carotenoids are found in foods that are yellow, orange, or red, like beets, carrots, peaches, apricots, tomatoes, pumpkin, peppers, oranges, and butternut squash. Even some green vegetables have high carotene content: spinach, kale, and turnip greens.

Another important reason to get enough carotenoids in your diet is that lack of vitamin A may be involved in the development of cervical cancer! We know human papillomavirus causes warts. Children sometimes get warts on their fingers; these warts are harmless and usually go away on their own. Papillomavirus can also infect the genital area, causing genital warts. Certain strains of the genital variety of the virus can cause your cells to become cancerous over time. Women who have cervical cancer from infection with human papillomavirus have low levels of vitamin A in their blood. Are women with low levels of vitamin A more prone to infection with human papillomavirus? Who knows! No scientist will go so far as to say that taking carotenoids, which your body will convert into vitamin A, will prevent cervical cancer, and neither will I. It does, however, seem prudent to eat plenty of red, orange, and yellow fruits and vegetables.

Folic acid is another important supplement. A deficiency of folic acid, a vitamin in the B family of vitamins, while you're pregnant can cause problems with the development of the baby's spinal cord. Most cereals and wheat products are fortified with folic acid, which is the man-made variety of folate, as are prenatal vitamins. Yet even folic acid has two sides to the story. It helps prevent colon cancer, but if you already have colon cancer and take high doses of folic acid, the tumors may grow more quickly! You may prefer to get your folate from natural sources: lentils, black beans, asparagus, and spinach. High doses of spinach have never been associated with the development of cancer.

Calcium is another supplement you should consider starting at age forty, thirty, or even twenty, *if and only if* you do not get enough in your diet. If you get plenty of calcium in your diet, calcium supplements will not give you anything more, except maybe kidney stones.

Cheese and milk are far and away the foods with the highest calcium content. Broccoli, kale, turnip greens, and tofu also have calcium, but not nearly as much as milk, cheese, and yogurt. If you're lactose intolerant and cannot drink milk or eat cheese, you probably aren't getting enough calcium in your diet and should take a supplement. You may also need a calcium supplement if you take prednisone for asthma or if you have been a lifelong soda drinker, as soda, especially cola, leaches calcium from your bones. If you went through menopause early, you're at especially high risk for osteoporosis. Estrogen is the key for calcium metabolism and bone formation in women. When you go through menopause, your estrogen level goes down and you start losing bone mass rapidly. If you never developed good strong bones when you were young, you do not have a big storehouse to lose when you go through menopause. You need your storehouse to be full so that when you lose some, your spine doesn't become bent over like the hunchback of Notre Dame.

It's probably too late for you to worry about how much bone you made when you were eighteen, so the best you can do now is keep what you have. You can, however, make sure your daughters get adequate calcium and vitamin D and get them out to exercise. Bones need a workout to get stronger. If you are going to take a calcium supplement, take five or six hundred milligrams twice a day with food. Taking it with food helps absorption. If you find the calcium supplement makes you sleepy, take one only with your evening meal. If it makes you constipated, skip it and get your calcium from food. The following list of calcium-rich foods should give you an idea of what to eat (calcium content is shown in milligrams):

> Beans, white (navy or cannellini), 1 cup: 191
> Beet greens, cooked and drained, 1 cup: 164
> Cabbage, Chinese (bok choy), 1 cup: 158
> Cheese, blue, 1 oz: 150
> Cheese, cheddar, 1 oz: 204
> Cheese, cottage, 1 cup: 126
> Cheese, cottage, 2% milk fat, 1 cup: 156
> Cheese, cottage, nonfat, 1 cup: 46
> Cheese, Muenster, 1 oz: 203
> Cheese, ricotta, part skim, 1 cup: 669
> Cheese, swiss, 1 oz: 204
> Collard greens, boiled and drained, 1 cup: 266
> Dandelion greens, boiled and drained, 1 cup: 147
> Milk, whole, 2%, 1%, or skim, 1 cup: 300
> Molasses, blackstrap, 2 Tbsp: 400
> Mustard greens, boiled and drained, 1 cup: 104
> Okra, boiled and drained, 1 cup: 123
> Okra, frozen, boiled, and drained, 1 cup: 177
> Spinach, boiled and drained, 1 cup: 245
> Turnip greens, boiled and drained, 1 cup: 197
> Yogurt, 8 oz: 400

Who would have ever thought that molasses was high in calcium? This list shows something else if you look closely. Nonfat milk products have low calcium content. Nonfat cottage cheese not only tastes disgusting, but is also low in calcium. So why eat that stuff?

Calcium alone isn't sufficient to prevent osteoporosis. Bones need a whole slew of nutrients, like magnesium, protein, and vitamin K, to stay strong. Magnesium is found in dark green leafy vegetables, like spinach, and in whole grains and nuts. Vitamin K is found in broccoli and dark green leafy vegetables. Now we have another reason to eat dark green leafy vegetables: bone health.

Calcium, along with vitamin D, may also help prevent "middle-age spread." One very large study showed that middle-aged women, if they weren't getting enough calcium or vitamin D from food in the first place, lost a little bit of weight when they took supplements.[2] The women not taking the calcium-plus-vitamin-D supplement gained weight. Other studies have shown that one or two servings of dairy products every day helps promote weight loss.[3] Sounds like a plan to me! Let me stress this again because it's so important: calcium from foods is a thousand times better than calcium from a supplement. All right, I'm exaggerating, but only slightly. If you look at the bone densities of women who get their calcium from food and compare them to the bone densities of women who get their calcium from supplements, the women who get their calcium from food have much stronger bones than the women taking high-dose calcium supplements, even though the women on supplements were getting twice as much calcium![4] Calcium from food is so much better for you.

2. B. Caan and others, "Calcium Plus Vitamin D Supplementation and the Risk of Postmenopausal Weight Gain," *Archives of Internal Medicine* 167, no. 9 (2007): 893–902.
3. National Dairy Council, "Dairy's Role in a Healthy Weight," http://www.nationaldairycouncil.org/NationalDairyCouncil/Healthyweight/Science.htm.
4. N. Napoli and others, "Effects of Dietary Calcium Compared with Calcium Supplements on Estrogen Metabolism and Bone Mineral Density," *American Journal of Clinical Nutrition* 85, no. 5 (2007): 1428–1433.

Is it ever that easy, though? No! There has been some new data released from a big study on calcium supplements. This new study showed that women who took calcium supplements had a higher risk of heart attacks![5] How could this be? No one expected this. There are some parts of the country where the water supply is rich in calcium. People who live in these areas have fewer heart attacks. To support this notion that calcium improves heart health, some large studies have shown fewer heart attacks in women who took calcium supplements. But this new study showed an increase in heart attacks. So which is right? Do calcium pills increase, or decrease your chances of having a heart attack? No one knows for sure, but this is another example proving to you that a pill can never take the place of healthy food, with two exceptions: vitamin D and folic acid during pregnancy. Vitamin D is so important that it gets its own chapter.

Aside from women who may become pregnant or are pregnant, whether to take a supplement is completely up to you. (Women who want to become pregnant should start their prenatal vitamins *before* they get pregnant.) But you could spend hundreds of dollars every month on multivitamins, calcium, fish oil capsules, fat burners, muscle builders, antioxidants, baldness cures, anticellulite pills, and anything else you could think of. Save your money. Do not buy any supplements yet.

Two women who work at our clinic asked the nutritionist for advice on what nutritional supplements to take. They wanted to lose a bit of weight, but more importantly, they wanted to be healthy and avoid developing diabetes. Our nutritionist, Olga, is fabulous; she is full of energy, is always happy, and eats healthier than anyone I know. So Olga provided them with a list of supplements to buy. A very good list indeed, with antioxidants, fish oil, flax, carnitine, and a few other supplements for fat burning and

5. M. J. Bolland and others, "Vascular Events in Healthy Older Women Receiving Calcium Supplementation: Randomized Controlled Trial," *BMJ* 336, no. 7638 (2008): 262–266.

overall health. The women spent $160 each for a one-month sup-
ply of the items on the list. If you have that kind of money to
spend, go for it. If not, your money is better spent on healthy fresh
fruits and vegetables.

When you're ready to buy supplements, you do not need to buy
everything at once. Start with a fish oil or omega-3-containing supplement. Take one of these on days when you aren't eating fish or putting
flaxseed oil on your salad. Better yet, buy cod-liver oil. All those generations of grandmothers knew what they were doing. How many of
you were given cod-liver oil when you were growing up? My patients
who were given Cod-liver oil as children say they never got sick. Cod-
liver oil has vitamin D, vitamin A, and omega-3 fatty acids.

I also highly recommend buying some of the powdered green
fruit and vegetable extracts to add to your morning power shake.
These powdered green foods have the phytonutrient equivalent of
five servings of fruits and vegetables. If you add one to your shake
in the morning, you'll start the day with a bang. It's better to start
your day with a power shake than with an artery-clogging, mind-
numbing Sausage McMuffin.

First, you need to choose a powdered extract. I've tried them
all. They are all equal, more or less. Some have a bit of a bitter
edge to them, especially the ones heavy on greens like wheat grass.
Some are sweeter, especially if they have more fruits. Some are
more expensive, some less expensive. Whichever one you choose,
refrigerate or freeze it after opening the jar. For a list of these green
vegetable extracts, see appendix 7.

For those of you on a budget, the shake is going to be the most
expensive thing you "eat" every day. Between the cost of the powdered green extract, the milk, the frozen blueberries, the peanut
butter, and the protein powder, it ends up costing close to four
dollars per serving. Compare that to a buttered roll with margarine, which only costs fifty cents at the corner bodega. If you save
money by avoiding weight-loss supplements, maybe you could
spend that money on your breakfast shake.

Most of the *weight-loss* supplements out there cost a hundred dollars a month or more. There is the Brazilian magic weight-loss pill, the Hoodia magic weight-loss pill, and the belly fat pill. There is even a magic weight-loss earring! Save your money. Appetite suppressants do suppress your appetite, but your body isn't stupid. It knows when it's starving. When you take the pill, it will curb your appetite. When the pill wears off, you'll be hungry. Your body will send signals to your brain, "I'm starving! I'm starving! Feed me! Feed me!" You certainly cannot control the urge to scratch an itch. Do you really expect to resist the urge to eat when you're hungry? Then you'll grab anything that isn't nailed down to stuff in your mouth. Even if you take the appetite suppressants every day for a year and lose a lot of weight, your body will rebel eventually.

Everybody knows somebody who lost a lot of weight using an appetite suppressant. What do these friends look like now? Right! They look exactly the same now as they did *before* they started the magic weight-loss pills. They gained back all of the weight, and then some. The only diets that work over the long haul are the ones where you eat enough so that you are not hungry, the ones with plenty of healthy, nutritious foods that also stress exercise or an active lifestyle. Healthy food and an active lifestyle: that's what works in the long run. Here is a good analogy. People think they can go on a diet for a month or two with the help of a supplement, and then go back to their old eating habits. That's like doing a big spring cleaning in April and then expecting the house to stay clean for the next year, or two years, or ten years. To keep your house clean, you need to be vigilant and do a little something every day. To keep your body healthy, you need to give it healthy nutritious food every day and get out and get moving.

If you have money to spare and want to buy some supplements, there are some I would recommend. These are supplements backed by scientific data in humans and animals. These are studies done by scientists who are not on the payroll of some fly-by-night vitamin company. These are studies duplicated by other scientists to ensure that the results are real. I'd like to see the double-blind, placebo-controlled trials of the Brazilian magic weight-loss pill. Those studies probably do not exist.

CLA, L-carnitine, omega-3 fatty acids, and vitamin D are supplements that have been shown, in study after study, to improve athletic performance and the body's ability to heal itself, and just generally improve a person's health and well-being. But wait to spend money on supplements. If you can, buy one of those powdered green fruit and vegetable extracts to put in your morning shake. By far, the most important thing to do is to spend your money on good healthy fruits and vegetables.

Chapter Seventeen

Let The Sun Shine In: Vitamin D

I f the only thing you learn from this book is the importance of vitamin D, it will have been a success. Vitamin D is essential for more than just bone health. Fifty years ago, scientists noticed that people who lived in the southern part of America had lower blood pressure than people living in the northern part. They figured it had something to do with sunshine, and so more studies were done. The bottom line, they found, is that people who are vitamin D deficient have higher blood pressure. If you give high doses of vitamin D to people who are deficient, when the vitamin D level in their blood becomes normal, their blood pressure comes down by an average of 9 percent. That may not seem like a lot, but it's a significant improvement. If, instead of a study of a vitamin, this was a study of a new blood pressure pill made by a big drug company, the price of the stock would have soared. The CEO would have gotten a big fat bonus and bought himself a brand new yacht. Instead, a vitamin gets no rave reviews at all. For some people, a 9 percent decrease in blood pressure means they no longer need a blood pressure medication.

And that's not all vitamin D does. Those researchers from fifty years ago also noticed that more people died of certain cancers in the North than in the South. Death rates for breast cancer, prostate cancer, and colon cancer are higher in the North than in the South. Again, they figured it had something to do with sunshine, and therefore vitamin D. In fact, vitamin D is the only vitamin I give to my boyfriend. Getting his vitamin D level to 70 ng/ml (nanograms/milliliter, also abbreviated µg/ml) will cut his chances of getting colon cancer by 75 percent.

Vitamin D also has an effect on glucose metabolism. It will not cure your diabetes, but if you have prediabetes and are vitamin D deficient, there might be some hope. Replacing your vitamin D might actually help prevent you from progressing to full-blown diabetes.

Vitamin D has an effect on the immune system as well. There may be an association between vitamin D deficiency and autoimmune diseases such as rheumatoid arthritis, multiple sclerosis, and type 1 (juvenile) diabetes.

Do you see a trend here? Diabetes, hypertension, breast cancer, prostate cancer, and colon cancer are all diseases associated with people of color. These same diseases are associated with vitamin D deficiency. People of color make less vitamin D and are more likely to be vitamin D deficient. As with vitamin A and cervical cancer, I will not tell you that taking vitamin D will prevent breast cancer, prostate cancer, or colon cancer. It will not prevent diabetes. It will not cure your hypertension. But it just seems prudent to make sure your vitamin D levels are adequate.

First, go get your level checked at your physician's office. Your physician can check your vitamin D levels for you with an easy and inexpensive blood test. Don't go by the "normal range" listed on the lab sheet. That "normal" range is based on the results of other people who are checking their vitamin D levels at the same lab. If everyone is deficient, the normal range at the lab will be low. Anything under 20 ng/ml is deficient or insufficient. 30 ng/ml is just at the border of acceptable. Many believe a blood level of 70 ng/ml is optimal. Anything over 100 ng/ml is overkill but not dangerous over the short term.

One of my patients had a blood level greater than 150 ng/ml. It was off the charts, higher than the upper limits of sensitivity of the test! I panicked, thinking I had given him a prescription for vitamin D and was overdosing him. Well, wasn't I surprised to find I had never given him a vitamin D prescription? He wasn't taking over-the-counter vitamin D either. He wasn't drinking cod-liver oil or eating sardines. He was just getting a lot of sunshine. Since then, I've seen this over and over in my patients who get a lot of sunshine. Their level of vitamin D is very high, from working outdoors, playing baseball on the weekends, or by traveling to the Caribbean to visit relatives twice a year. This goes to show you: we really do not know what our level of vitamin D would be if we spent as much time outdoors, running around naked, as nature intended us to.

If you are deficient, you can supplement yourself, under your physician's supervision, with one to two thousand international units (IUs) a day, or ten thousand IUs once a week, until your levels are normal. You cannot use wimpy doses of vitamin D if you need to replace your stores. It might take awhile, a few months even. Go back to your doctor, and get your level rechecked to see how it's coming along. And don't forget, the lifestyle that made you deficient will make you deficient again. You may need to take a vitamin D supplement every day for life.

If you need to get aggressive with your vitamin D replacement, you can obtain a prescription for a fifty-thousand-IU pill you take once or twice a week. Do not do this aggressive, high-dose replacement without the very close supervision of your physician. Although fifty thousand IUs sounds like an astronomical dose, it's safe for those who are very deficient.

Some patients ask about the little cod-liver-oil pills that have been sold in pharmacies for the past fifty years. Cod-liver oil is an excellent source of vitamin D, but you need to get the liquid oil, not the pills. Yes, I know what you're thinking: yuck. If you want to get the cod-liver-oil pills, read the label on the jar. There simply is not enough vitamin D in the little pills to replenish your stores. You also need to read the bottle of cod-liver oil. Some brands do not have very much vitamin D per tablespoon. You'd have to overdose on the vitamin A content in order to get enough vitamin D. Since you might need a very large daily dose to reverse a vitamin D deficiency, you're better off getting a prescription. You can buy vitamin D capsules containing one or two thousand IUs, but anything over two thousand IUs is by prescription only. After your stores are replaced, you can switch to the over-the-counter pills or to cod-liver oil. Milk is fortified with vitamin D, but not enough for adults. Children drink a lot of milk. If milk were fortified with enough vitamin D for adults, children would be overdosed.

There are some foods that are great sources of vitamin D as seen in this chart:[1]

Food	International Units Per Serving
Cod-liver oil, 1 tablespoon	1,360
Salmon, cooked, 3 ½ ounces	360
Mackerel, cooked, 3 ½ ounces	345
Tuna fish, canned in oil, 3 ounces	200
Sardines, canned in oil, drained, 1 ¾ ounces	250
Orange juice, fortified with vitamin D, 8 ounces	100
Milk, fortified with vitamin D, 8 ounces	100

Get creative with these sources of vitamin D. The Spanish make a type of tapas with sardines. Tapas are those little appetizers served

1. Office of Dietary Supplements, "Dietary Supplement Fact Sheet: Vitamin D," National Institutes of Health, http://ods.od.nih.gov/factsheets/vitamind.asp.

in bars and restaurants all across Spain. The skinless and boneless variety may be the way to go when making this treat. Taking the bones and tail off of every sardine in a can is a messy and smelly process. Either way, open a can of sardines, and put it on a healthy whole grain cracker. Pretend you're sitting in a tapas bar in Madrid while you enjoy them. Italians make a pasta dish with sardines sautéed with onions and garlic. Another trick is to pour one tablespoon of cod-liver oil on your salad every day. It does give a fishy flavor to your salad, though, so pretend you're eating a Caesar salad (anchovies give the dressing its intense flavor). If you happen to love anchovies, cod-liver oil on your salad will be a delicious treat. Expand your horizons. You'll never go back to McDonald's again.

You don't need to get your vitamin D from food or supplements. Our bodies can make up to the equivalent of four or five thousand IUs of vitamin D every day. We may even be able to make as much as ten thousand IUs every day, under the right conditions. Still, very few of us get enough sunshine to make our daily requirement of vitamin D. We avoid the sun. We use sunscreen. We cover up with hats. We work indoors. We just aren't getting enough sunshine.

People who are pale need less sunshine to make vitamin D. People of color need more because less of the sun's rays get through to the inner layers of the skin, where vitamin D is made. During the winter, forget about it! No one makes enough vitamin D in the winter.

You don't need a lot of sunshine to make your daily requirement of vitamin D. Just ten to thirty minutes of direct sunshine over 50 percent of your body every day will do it. More if you're dark skinned, less if you're light skinned. More during the winter, less during the summer. More if you live in Maine, less if you live in Florida.

Forget the sunscreen. UVB makes vitamin D. Most sunscreens block both UVA and UVB rays of the sun. Even a sunscreen with an SPF of eight will block 85 percent of the sun's rays. A good rule

of thumb is that as soon as you start to get a faint hint of color…
stop. You are done. You have even gone too far. You've made your
vitamin D for the day, and it's time to run, cover up, put on the
hat, and break out the sunscreen. Do not get red. Do not get burnt.
More is not better. First of all, vitamin D production stops at about
four thousand to ten thousand IUs for the day. Second, the skin has
a built-in "off" switch. As soon as you've gone too far, vitamin D
production turns off as the body tries to protect itself.

Don't overdo the sunshine. A few years back, a group of us
went to a resort in the Dominican Republic to celebrate the for-
tieth birthday of a friend. There were ten or twelve of us. One
woman in the group had incredible skin. Not a mark. No ugly
cellulite. No heartbreaking psoriasis. Not even one varicose vein or
broken blood vessel on her legs. No tan lines broke up the perfectly
even color of her complexion. You know how your chest and arms
get darker than your legs. Not this woman! Her skin was perfect.

The way she kept her skin flawless was by staying huddled
under a big umbrella, wearing a hat and a long-sleeved blouse. It
was ninety-nine degrees outside, and she was wearing a long-sleeved
blouse! Any body part not covered with clothes was smeared with
thick, white zinc oxide sunscreen. She is living proof that women
can keep their skin young by avoiding the sun. Just be sure to get
enough vitamin D through food or supplements.

Chapter Eighteen

The Diet: When Fat, Fit, and Fabulous Is Not Enough

So what's going on here? *Where's the diet?* You're probably saying to yourself, "All I have so far is a list of foods to avoid that contain either trans fats or HFCS, and a proclamation to eat ten servings of fruits and vegetables every day."

"I get to put olive oil on my salad and eat a handful of nuts every day, but I need to cut way down on my starches and replace them with complex carbohydrates."

"I should never go hungry."

"I need to make new friends who are into health and fitness, and I need to get out and move."

"I do not need to spend money on special foods or supplements, but I might need to take a vitamin D supplement."

"And I get to eat chocolate!"

Not much of a diet! Maybe not, but you could stop right here and live a very healthy life. You'd stop gaining weight. You'd probably lose weight, especially if you are exercising. You're headed to a new set-point weight for the amount you eat and the amount you exercise. If you are happy, you can stop right here. Isn't this great?

This is not a diet about deprivation. It's about lifestyle changes. It's about health and happiness. Worry about your health, not about your weight.

My recommendation *is* to stop right here. Eat your five to ten servings of fruits and vegetables every day. Limit the starches. Eliminate the HFCS and trans fats. Increase your intake of healthy fats and get some exercise. See what weight your body gravitates to. Give it a little time: a couple of weeks or a couple of months. If you hit a plateau and aren't happy with your body, then you know it's time to make more changes. Maybe it's time to cut back on the starches a bit more, exercise more vigorously, or eat less. You might need to get serious and count calories. Counting calories is a big pain in the neck, no doubt about it. Other diets like Weight Watchers and Atkins count points. If you're having trouble achieving your goals, you may need to count something.

If counting calories or counting points isn't for you, don't stress over it. With the changes you've made, you're living a healthy lifestyle. You may not be skinny, but you are healthy.

Chapter Nineteen

Meal Choices

Patients always want me to tell them what to eat. That's difficult because it all depends on what is in season, what is on sale, and what you're in the mood for. It also depends on what you have cooked and ready to go when it's mealtime. Most importantly, it depends on your cultural heritage. Someone of Mexican descent might never eat dandelion greens, but will eat verdolaga. A woman of Puerto Rican ancestry might not try arugula, but remembers eating watercress as a child. So interpret these meal choices in the context of your culinary heritage. These are a few examples, some for hot weather and some for cold weather. These are real-world ideas because I work, I am busy, and I have to go to the supermarket just like you do. These are practical ideas.

Sometimes I read a two-week diet plan from another book and realize the writer is not living on the same planet as we are. Here is an example of one day of a seven-day diet my sister found:

Breakfast:
3 egg white omelet with
2 oz. chopped ham

1 oz. swiss cheese

1 cup cantaloupe

Snack:

¾ cup 2% cottage cheese

1 cup strawberries

1 tablespoon chopped walnuts

Lunch:

2 cups salad greens

4 oz. grilled chicken

2 tablespoons low-fat dressing

1 orange

Snack:

1 apple

2 tablespoons hummus

Dinner:

4 oz. grilled halibut

1 cup sautéed spinach with 1 teaspoon olive oil

Mixed green salad with 2 tablespoons low-fat dressing

What's wrong with this diet? Each day was a variation on this same theme. Every day had vegetables and protein, two snacks, some nuts. The diet is a bit low in essential fatty acids and omega-3s. It's a bit low in calcium, so you'd have to take a supplement. But it's really not a bad diet. I'd starve on it. You'd probably starve on it too.

I'll tell you what's really wrong with this diet! Who goes out and buys two tablespoons of hummus? No! You have to buy a whole sixteen-ounce container. What are you going to do with the leftover hummus? It's going to sit in your refrigerator and grow green, fuzzy mold. How do you go out and buy four ounces of halibut? This is just not a diet for the real world.

So let's do a few menus for each season: soups in the winter, salads in the summer, and vegetables in season. Realize you are going to be cooking. Set aside half a day each week to shop and prepare. You'll be washing vegetables and salads. Realize you'll be eating leftovers. You will need to make extra food in order to pack a lunch for work. Realize you will be eating the same foods for a couple of days in a row, maybe even longer. Do I hear some complaints from the peanut gallery about eating the same leftovers two or three days in a row? Did you ever complain about eating ice cream every night? Potato chips every night? Hamburgers and french fries every day for lunch? Rice and beans every night for dinner? Do not complain about eating the same healthy foods a couple of days in a row. You've eaten the same high-fat, high-starch, high-sugar, brain-fog foods for a few weeks in a row, if not for months or years in a row. Why not eat the same healthy foods for a few days in a row then?

In broad brushstrokes, you'll see a trend. Three meals and two snacks. Many meals do not contain meat. Replace meat with beans or legumes a few meals every week. You'll see every day includes some sort of green leafy vegetable. Nuts are eaten every day, usually as a snack. There are no sugary desserts. Those are not on the program, except as a rare treat. Fruit should be your dessert, preferably grapes when they are in season. If you pay attention to the news, you may have heard about resveratrol. It's an antioxidant found in grapes and may contribute to a longer life.

In appendix 2, there are more ideas for meal choices, but here are a few:

Breakfast:

Blueberry-green shake (See the recipe section. Not exactly Mediterranean, but healthy.)

Or

One cup oatmeal plus one or two links of chicken sausage or two eggs (It's best to use the slow-cooking, steel-cut oatmeal, since it has GLA, one of the essential fatty acids. Make a big pot the night before, with cinnamon and a handful of raisins for flavor. Sprinkle some chopped pecans or walnuts on top for added crunch. Split it into four one-cup servings. That way, you have oatmeal ready for four days in a row.)

Or

Scrambled eggs or an omelet, and some fruit

Snack (The same ideas can be used for the midmorning or afternoon snacks.):

Chicken fingers and a can of V8 juice

Or

Handful of nuts and a piece of fruit or a can of V8 juice

Or

Guacamole dip with carrot sticks and sliced cucumber for dipping

Or

Dry-popped popcorn, up to ten cups (This is a great late-night snack if you like to nosh at night and need something crunchy.)

Or

If you're serious about going Mediterranean all the way, have olives with radishes and a sliced red bell pepper on the side.

Lunch:

Nicoise salad (just a fancy French name for a can of tuna with some olives on a bed of lettuce)

Or

Split pea soup

Or

Plain yogurt topped with fruit, walnuts, and granola

Dinner (Any of the lunch ideas can be used for dinner as well.):

Lamb chops, a baked sweet potato or butternut squash, dandelion greens sautéed in olive oil, and fruit for dessert

Or

Steak, a baked potato, asparagus with lemon, and a tomato
salad

Or

Spinach and bean soup (See recipe section.)

Or

Salmon, sautéed Swiss chard, two-thirds cup wild rice, and
artichoke heart salad

Does that sound like a lot of food? It sure is. Compare that to
your old eating habits. A typical breakfast for you might be a Sausage McMuffin with Egg at 450 calories. Instead, for a total of 460
calories, you could eat:

1. one cup oatmeal with one tablespoon brown sugar
   and a few raisins at 200 calories;

2. two hard-boiled eggs with the yolks at 160
   calories;

3. one orange at 100 calories.

You'd be absolutely satisfied after that healthy breakfast, but
still hungry after one Sausage McMuffin with Egg. One of those
just doesn't do it for me. Theoretically, it should. It has plenty of
calories and fat, but I'm still hungry after eating one. You should
borrow the documentary *Super Size Me* from the library. It will be
a real eye-opener.

Chapter Twenty

For Men Only

One of my male diabetic patients felt that there was not enough information for men in this book. Men do not typically go to the bookstore to buy diet books, so this chapter is for the men who might be reading their wife's, sister's, girlfriend's, or mother's copy of this book.

First, let's work on some motivation. For every 30 pounds a man is overweight, the penis becomes one inch shorter. This is because of the structure of the fat pad in the lower pelvis. If that isn't motivation enough, as men gain fat weight, the levels of hormones change. Everyone knows testosterone is the male hormone. It's the hormone that surges when a boy goes through puberty and causes him to develop male sexual characteristics. It's the hormone that determines how high someone's sex drive is. Testosterone makes men look like men, and not like women. Testosterone gives a man a male outlook on life with determination and drive. It's "the male hormone." Estrogen, the "the female hormone," is exactly the opposite. It's what makes women soft and feminine.

Well, everyone, men and women, has both testosterone and estrogen. Women just have a lot more estrogen, and men have a lot more testosterone. In the body, estrogen and testosterone are actually converted back and forth, from one to the other. This occurs in the liver and *in fat tissue*. In men who are of normal weight, this is in perfect and delicate balance, with testosterone ruling at the end of the day. In men who are overweight, too much of their testosterone is converted into estrogen. What happens to those men with too much estrogen? First of all, their muscles become flabby. Not all men need to be like Rambo, but a man should be able to do a couple of push-ups.

After your muscles become flabby, the estrogen starts to stimulate growth of the breasts. They have a very unflattering nickname, which cannot be repeated in polite company. Not only is breast enlargement in men unsightly, but it also puts a man at an increased risk of breast cancer.

The extra weight increases one's chances of developing diabetes and hypertension. These two diseases destroy the blood vessels that engorge the penis with blood for an erection. Relationships suffer. All the Viagra in the world cannot help if the blood vessels are damaged.

Most importantly, though, men with young male children need to set an example for the little ones. Boys want to be just like their dads. If Dad is a couch potato, then that's what Junior aspires to be too. Young boys with excess fat have too much estrogen and too little testosterone. The excess estrogen interferes with their normal male sexual development during puberty. And it will be your fault because you were too busy eating and sitting on the couch, watching TV.

So here is a short list of things you can do to start turning your health around and to inspire your children to be healthy too:

☐ Involve the whole family in physical activity. Instead of buying the children video games as holiday presents, purchase soccer balls, tennis rackets, bikes, or equipment for any sport that strikes their fancy. If that's too expensive, even a Frisbee will do.

Then, you need to take the children out and teach them how to play. There is a ball field near my house, and it's always full of fathers and sons playing ball together. What a wonderful way to bond. And it's a wonderful way for your son to burn off all his extra energy.

☐ Eat your vegetables, especially green leafy vegetables like spinach. Yes, real men don't eat vegetables, but you have the power to change America one family at a time. You're setting an example for your children.

☐ Stop drinking soda, juice, iced tea, or any sweetened soft drink. Sweet drinks are stored in the belly as fat. This belly fat is associated with the development of diabetes.

☐ Don't skip meals, and don't go hungry. People who miss meals tend to overeat at the next meal.

☐ Eat healthy snacks in between meals. Nuts are an especially healthy snack. Not only do they curb your hunger, but they may also help prevent heart attacks.

☐ Cut down on the starches for the same reason you need to stop drinking soda or other sweetened drinks. Overdoing the starches can pack on the pounds, especially in the belly.

Your family needs you. Please try to stay healthy! As I asked our housewife friend in chapter 3, what do you want on your gravestone? "Beloved son, husband, and father. He loved to eat and watch TV." Or would you prefer it to be engraved with, "Beloved son, husband, and father. He was a great inspiration to us all."

Chapter Twenty-one

Do These Shoes Make Me Look Fat?

S hould you wear the stiletto heels or the Birkenstock orthopedic sandals? Do you choose the stilettos, even if you can't walk in them? Aha! Another fashion victim, guilty as charged!

Here in New York City, where everyone walks a lot, you see beautiful young women walking down the street all the time. Their hair is shiny and perfectly coiffed. They are wearing fancy designer duds and carrying the newest "it" purse. Their legs are firm and shapely from yoga and kickboxing, with three-inch Manolo Blahnik shoes on their perfectly pedicured feet. But what is wrong with their faces? Why aren't they smiling? Why are their faces scrunched up like they just ate a lemon ball? Their feet hurt, that's why. They're probably hungry too.

Social researchers did a poll of parents about their views on children. Overwhelmingly, parents preferred a child with a learning disability to a child who is fat. Surveys of the obese have shown they would rather be blind or lose a leg than be obese. This tells us how deep the discrimination toward fat people goes. Do you wear painful uncomfortable shoes and clothes because you think they make you look thinner? More beautiful?

My mother was always watching her weight. Even when she was in her eighties, she worried she was too fat. She wanted to lose ten pounds. Believe me, she was just fine. Why would an eighty-three-year-old woman at a perfect weight worry she was too fat?

Our society is superficial and judgmental, so much so that parents would rather have a child with a learning disability than a weight problem. How do we go about changing a society that has gotten lost?

I have a couple of ideas. Nothing based in science or backed by research. It's just some advice based on years of taking care of patients. First of all, rebel! You already are fabulous and beautiful. You just need to figure out how to feel beautiful on the inside. Start by standing up straight and walking down the street like you own it.

Next, we need to take a cue from our sexy sisters in France, Italy, Spain, and South America. They still eat together as a family. Dinner is about socializing, conversation, and communication. In his book *The Fat Fallacy*, Dr. Will Clower writes about his experiences living in France. He writes about the French people, their relationship with food, and what he learned living among the French. One of the French scientists he worked with told him the reason Americans eat so much is because we are starving emotionally. He is right. Go to any restaurant. Watch families or couples eating together. No one is laughing. No one is talking. No one is communicating. Everybody is just shoveling food into his or her mouth. The point is that you do not eat mindlessly if the focus of the meal is removed from the food and placed on the person you are eating with.

Food has to be about life and love. Food needs to be nurturing. It cannot be a crutch or a substitute because food can never satisfy an emotional void. Eat when you are hungry, not when you are lonely. Get in touch with your inner hunger because food can never fill a hole in your heart.

Chapter Twenty-two

In Conclusion

Putting it all together, this is nothing new to you:

Stop drinking soda.

Spread your food out throughout the day in three meals and one to two snacks.

Exercise.

Avoid trans fats.

Increase your intake of healthy fats.

Avoid foods made with high fructose corn syrup.

Eat at least five servings of fruits and vegetables every day.

Eat a dark green leafy vegetable every day.

Organize your life and your kitchen.

Cut way down on the starches you eat.

Get some sunshine, or take a vitamin D supplement.

Eat when you are hungry.

Sleep when you are tired.

Stand up straight and walk down the street like you own it, with a smile on your face, knowing you are living a life that is healthy, vital, and fulfilled. You may or may not be fat according to the little BMI calculator. It does not matter, because you are fit and beautiful.

Chapter Twenty-three

Let's Cook

The first thing you need to do before you start cooking is organize your kitchen. Get the clutter and chaos out of your life and out of your kitchen. Several years ago, I moved from Washington, DC, back to New York City. Well, all the horror stories you hear about how expensive apartments are in New York City are true. So a friend graciously agreed to let me stay with her during the week while I was working during the day and apartment hunting in the evenings. The deal was that I would cook healthy meals and pack breakfast and lunch for her to take to work. Little did I know what I was getting into! In order to get to the sink, I had to move shopping bags of stuff out of the way. There were bags of empty cans and bottles waiting to go back to the supermarket. There were bags of groceries. There were bags of bags. There was a case of canned mandarin oranges. At least it could have been a case of sardines. There were so many magnets on the cabinet doors that if you tried to take a dish out, a magnet would go flying and start a chain reaction. There would be a cascade of stuff falling out of the dish drainer and off the counters onto the floor.

What's the moral of the story? If your kitchen sounds like my friend's kitchen, ask a few organized and ruthless friends (who are also good cooks) to come over. Everyone has a friend or two who are control freaks. When they are in your kitchen organizing and eliminating excess junk, relax. Leave them alone, and let them do their job. They will organize your kitchen so it's easier to cook in. In order to cook, you need to be able to easily reach for a spoon or a bowl.

As hard as it will be to part with your accumulated useless stuff, just do it. Stuff, like food, can never fill a hole in your heart.

Let's Outfit Your Kitchen

You'll need some kitchen essentials. If you only own aluminum pots and pans, go ahead and use them for now. You'll need to replace them slowly over time with cookware that does not leach toxic substances into your food. Stainless steel is excellent. Stainless steel pots and pans with copper bottoms are even better. Cast iron is great. Cast iron, when properly maintained, can be fairly nonstick. Nonstick pans are another story entirely. Many of the health food purists refuse to use nonstick pans. They are concerned about Teflon, which is a known carcinogen, getting into their food. I try not use nonstick pans, but sometimes I do, carefully making sure not to overheat the pan. If you have an oven that stays warm because of the pilot light, do not store your nonstick pans in there. The heat will cause some fumes to come off the pan. Especially do not put an empty nonstick pan on a burner to get hot before you add the oil or water for cooking. More fumes! Birds are very sensitive to these fumes. I read an article about some poor man whose parrot died from the fumes of an empty Teflon pan put on a burner to heat up. This might be one of those crazy, made-up stories that circulate on the Internet, like the story about spiders in the toilet of an airplane that bit passengers on the buttocks. Whether or not the parrot story is true, we need to be careful when using nonstick pans.

Throw out your Teflon pans if they are getting scratched, making little flakes of Teflon come off onto your food. That's a good way to get cancer! And for Heaven's sake, do not use metal forks to turn foods in your nonstick pans. That's a good way to scratch the nonstick surface.

Even though I'm talking about Teflon-coated pans, there are all sorts of new types of nonstick cookware available. These new nonstick pans are coated with chemicals with names like perfluorooctane sulfonate and perfluorooctanoate. Do you really think these are any safer than Teflon? There have been some recent studies that have shown that women with the highest level of these chemicals in their blood have babies with slightly lower birth weights. Over time, one at a time, get some decent stainless steel and cast-iron pans. They will last a lifetime.

People like to use nonstick pans because they are nonstick. It doesn't take a genius to figure that out. Your stainless steel and cast-iron pans should not be sticking either! If your food is sticking in your stainless steel pots and pans, it's either because you're not using enough oil, the flame is too high, or even worse, because the pans are not clean. If you don't scrupulously clean your pots and pans, when they dry, you'll see whitish discoloration around the rims and on the bottom. That's where the food sticks when you try to cook in a dirty pan. Use the special stainless steel or aluminum scouring powders, right next to the Ajax and Comet, in the supermarket. Soak the pans overnight if necessary, and use a little elbow grease. Your pots and pans should be spotless.

If you are new to cooking, you don't need a fancy set of twenty pots and pans. You'll see that you are using the same three or four pots and pans over and over.

Pots and Pans
One nine-inch or ten-inch sauté pan with a lid
One four-quart pot with a lid
One eight-quart pot with a lid

One very large pot to boil water, make soup, or cook big batches
   of green leafy vegetables
One fourteen-inch skillet
One roasting pan

Other Kitchen Essentials
Wooden spoons and spatulas:
> They will not scratch the bottom of your pans. There is
> never a reason to use a metal spoon to stir your food.
Blender for making shakes in the morning
Mixing bowls in three sizes: small, medium, and large
Lemon reamer or citrus squeezer:
> If you get a lemon reamer (which looks like an elongated
> top, the kind kids would spin in the old days, back when
> kids still went outside to play), do not get a plastic one.
> The plastic reamers slip and don't do a good job. Get a
> wooden one. If you *love* lemonade, save up to buy one of
> those hand-cranked, professional citrus presses. Making
> large batches of lemonade with a little reamer is a messy
> and tedious process, but with one of those presses, it's
> a breeze. One will set you back anywhere from $50 to
> $120. They're hard to find, and you may end up buying
> it on the Internet. You'll still need one of those little
> hand reamers for the times when you're only squeezing
> one or two lemons.
Sieves (colanders), for draining your vegetables, in three sizes:
   small, medium, and large
Salad spinner (optional):
> You could save twenty dollars, though, by using clean
> dishtowels instead. After washing your salad greens, let
> them drain in a sieve. Lay out a clean kitchen towel,
> not the fuzzy kind. Use something smooth and soft,
> like a flour sack towel. Flour sack towels are large, thin,
> cotton kitchen towels. Scatter the greens over the entire

towel. Next, roll up the towel gently, like a jellyroll, with the greens inside. Not too tight or else the greens will become bruised and get mushy. The towel absorbs the excess water. You could even store the entire roll in the refrigerator. The greens will stay fresh for days this way.

Vegetable peeler:

Do not skimp here. Buy one from Oxo Good Grips. They are more expensive but worth every penny.

Measuring cups:

Buy one set of metal ones for your dry measure and a large, heat-resistant, four-cup measuring cup.

Small bullet or mini-prep food processor:

The mini-prep food processors do a much better job at salad dressings and pesto than blenders do. If you have a large food processor, great! But if you're only making one cup of salad dressing, you certainly aren't going to be dragging out the big food processor. That's where the mini-prep comes in. I use my mini-prep all the time, but have never once used my big, fancy food processor. It's just taking up space in my cabinet. A mini-prep food processor will set you back around thirty dollars.

Sharp knives:

You'll need two or three good knives. Take care of them! Do not store them in a drawer, unless they are the only objects in that drawer, and they don't touch each other. Knives cannot clang against other things because it will dent the edges. Immediately after using your good knives, wash them and put them away. Do not throw them in the sink with all the other dirty dishes. That's how they get ruined. If you can get to a restaurant supply store, you can get decent knives with plastic handles for not that much money. I don't like knives with plastic handles. They feel a little slippery to me, especially if I'm cutting meat or if my hands are a little greasy. You can get high-quality, expensive knives that will last a lifetime by saving up and buying one good knife a year. You'd have a whole collection in no time, but you really don't need a whole collection. You really only need three knives: a small four-inch paring knife, a medium six-inch utility/sandwich knife, and a large eight- or nine-inch chef's knife—plus a steel rod or whetstone to sharpen them. Ask your butcher at the supermarket, or the fishmonger, to show you the hand motion to use to sharpen the knife on the whetstone. Stainless steel knives hold their edges longer, but if you have any old carbon steel knives from your grandmother, don't throw them out. They get very sharp, but they don't hold an edge. They need to be sharpened on the whetstone after every use.

Cleaver:

Don't spend a lot of money on a cleaver. The twenty-dollar cleavers they sell in Chinatown are better than the expensive ones. You'll need a cleaver to cut butternut and acorn squash in half. If you have no intention of ever making butternut or acorn squash, you will not need a cleaver.

Cast-iron frying pan(s):

Read the instructions on how to cure them. Basically, you spread a small amount of cooking oil on the new pan and stick it in a warm oven for a few hours. Cast-iron pans improve with age. Buy a good one. The cheaper ones have hot and cold spots and will not cook evenly. The extra money you spend will be worth it because these pans last forever. I have a cast-iron frying pan I inherited from my grandmother, and it still cooks perfectly. That pan must be seventy years old, or more; it was old when I was young, and I'm no spring chicken!

The one thing you must do, when you clean your cast-iron pan, is dry it immediately after you wash it. If you wipe it with a dishtowel, the dishtowel will become discolored. So don't dry cast iron with a dishtowel. Dry the pan on the stove over a flame. The purists never use water on their cast iron; they just wipe out the oil. My concern is that if you aren't using it every day, the oil will turn rancid, so I wash mine.

If you notice some rust stains on the bottom of your cast-iron pan, it's nothing. It just means the pan wasn't completely dry when you put it away. Just wash it again, and really get it dry before you put it away next time.

Long tongs:

It's much easier to turn certain foods, like vegetables or meats, with tongs than it is with a fork. There is never any reason to use a fork to turn your food when you cook.

Food scale (optional):

You'll need a small food scale if you plan on counting calories.

Calorie-counter book:

If you are going to count calories, you'll need a book that lists the fat and calorie content of various foods. You need this so you can see exactly what you are eating and why you are overweight. You'd be shocked at the calorie content of some of the foods you eat, and overeat.

Wooden cutting board or chopping block:

Don't get one that's too small or else you'll make more work for yourself in the long run.

Whisk (optional, but I use mine all the time; maybe you will too.)

Ladle big enough to dish out all the soup you're going to be making

Can opener

Microplane grater (optional):

This grater looks like a carpenter's rasp. The cutting teeth are very sharp and are excellent for zesting a lemon. If you never intend to zest a lemon, skip it.

Start buying these kitchen essentials one by one. Organize your kitchen. Clean out the clutter.

Now You're Ready to Cook

The first thing you need to do is go food shopping. Get the staples and buy vegetables. Green leafy vegetables won't last forever in the fridge. Don't store your leafy vegetables in plastic bags; otherwise, they will turn brown and mushy. Plan your vegetable shopping around your schedule. You need to make sure you have enough time to process the vegetables when you arrive home. You'll need to wash the green leafy vegetables, and then store them in a flour sack towel in the fridge. If you just throw the fresh vegetables in the fridge, you will never get around to cooking them.

Pick one half day every week to prepare meals. Turn on some music, or turn on the TV. Invite a friend over to keep you company while you cook; then, have dinner together. Involve the children in meal preparation, so they start learning how to cook.

Multitask! Make a big pot of split pea soup while you're making dinner. Then, you can freeze the soup in individual containers to take to work or use on another night. Cook two or three meals at once: a meal for today, a meal for tomorrow, and some extra meals to freeze for another day when you don't have time to cook.

Economize! Use the leftover bones from store-bought rotisserie chicken to make chicken or onion soup. One chicken carcass doesn't make much soup, so freeze the bones until you get enough to make a pot. Truthfully, the bones from a leftover rotisserie chicken do not make the best chicken soup, but you can use them for onion soup.

To save money, you can soak dried beans overnight to make a big pot of beans. Freeze the leftovers. There are so many ways to economize. Quit smoking if you smoke. That's close to $10 a day right there! Stop buying soda, and drink water. Buy bags of dry beans instead of cans. Rent movies from Blockbuster instead of going out to the movies. It doesn't matter if you see a movie the weekend it comes out, or if you wait until it comes out on video. Carry a bottle of water with you instead of buying one when you get to where you're going. Did you know a typical person who buys bottled water spends $1,200 per year on those bottles of water? If instead you put that money into a savings account every year, at 5 percent interest, you'd have $39,669 in the bank after twenty years. What would you do with $39,669? Not only that, but the empty bottles are clogging the landfills. Bottles of water are not good for your pocketbook nor for the environment. If there's a will, there's a way. You'll figure it out.

Plan ahead! Make double of everything, so you're not cooking every day. Make a pot of oatmeal, and pack individual one- or two-cup containers to warm up for breakfast. Bake sweet potatoes when you have the oven on for something else. If you want to drink a shake every morning for breakfast, have everything ready. It can take less than a minute to make a shake in the morning if everything has a place in your cabinets. It will be easy to grab the ingredients to throw together in the blender. Defrost your frozen fruit in the refrigerator the night before. Have containers of milk in the fridge, a clean to-go cup with a leakproof lid, and a box of straws ready. If you're a busy working mom, you'll need to be able to make your shake quickly and efficiently, so you can pack it up and take it to work in the morning.

Save time! Save money!

Chapter Twenty-four

Recipes

First a little background. These recipes are just as much about learning techniques as they are about a particular recipe. The *New York Times* interviewed Tom Colicchio, the head judge on *Top Chef*. When asked to name his most-used cookbook, he replied, "Recipes tell you nothing. Learning techniques is the key." And so, each recipe has a little preamble, explaining the technique for those of you who are new to cooking.

Almost all the recipes contain garlic, which is universal in the Mediterranean diet. An easy way to peel garlic is to lightly smash it with the flat side of a knife. To do this, lay the blade of the knife flat on a wooden chopping board. Put one clove under the wide part of the knife. (The handle has to be overhanging the edge of the board or else it will get in the way.) With your fist, carefully give the flat side of the knife a good whack, right over the spot with the clove. The paperlike cover of the garlic will come right off. The harder you whack the clove, the more mashed the garlic. It's your choice, depending on how mashed you like your garlic. You could pound the knife a few times and get the garlic really mashed. That would release more of the garlic flavor, but you need to be careful when you're cooking with the smashed garlic. The little bits will burn quickly.

When heating garlic, onions, or any vegetable in oil, do not wait until the oil is shimmering and smoking to add the vegetables. If you overheat the oil, you destroy the fragile essential fatty acids and start to create toxic by-products. You can add the garlic at the same time as you put the oil in the pan. Then, you heat both together. The garlic helps to prevent the oil from overheating. When the garlic starts to turn golden brown, which usually takes a minute or two, add the other vegetables. As a matter of fact, what real chefs do, and I am not one, is heat the pan first. When the pan is hot, they quickly add the oil and then the garlic.

Whatever you do, do not overcook vegetables. They aren't supposed to be mushy, soggy, or gray.

As we discussed previously, you don't need a lot of spices and herbs. The Mediterranean way is to use fresh vegetables, process them as little as possible, and let their flavors shine. Seriously, 90 percent of the time my vegetables are only seasoned with salt and pepper. No herbs. No spices. No sauces. If you use the coarse grain kosher salt and freshly ground black pepper, you'll see a big difference. On TV, the celebrity chefs give a quick twist or two of their pepper grinders. Let me tell you, it's a lie. A little dainty twist of the grinder isn't going to give you much pepper. Use some elbow grease, and really twist that grinder. Get some pepper on your food!

You won't find any meat recipes here. Cooking meat doesn't seem to be a problem for anyone. It's the vegetables everyone seems to have trouble with.

Vegetables

Here are a few of my favorite vegetable recipes. Some are quick and easy. Others are more involved. If you intend to try only one recipe from the selection, by all means, try the bitter greens in olive oil and garlic.

Bitter Greens with Garlic and Olive Oil

This is the most important recipe in this chapter. It's used all over the Mediterranean. Anyone from Greece or Italy will tell you these bitter, green leafy vegetables are the secret to good health.

A typical technique for cooking greens is to put a small amount of oil in the bottom of a big soup pot. Lightly brown garlic in the oil, and then add the vegetables. Let them cook down, and turn them with a long wooden spoon or tongs. You could do this with any green leafy vegetable: spinach, kale, collard greens, Swiss chard, dandelion greens, etc. Any of these can be cooked with this technique.

On TV, some chefs blanch the greens first in boiling water before sautéing in olive oil. Blanching is a cooking technique in which you quickly boil the greens. Then, you remove the greens from the boiling water and cool them quickly by plunging them into a bowl of ice water for a minute. The greens are removed from the ice water and drained for a minute on paper towels. The chef would then proceed with the garlic and olive oil sauté. This is absolutely unnecessary—it's a waste of time, a waste of energy, and makes extra dirty dishes and pots to wash. You can sauté the fresh greens directly in the oil.

There is a quick description of how to wash your leafy greens in the Wine, Chocolate, Lemons, and Parsley chapter. When the greens no longer have any grit or sand, let them drain. The longer you let them drain, the drier they will be when you cook them. The greens will give off water when you cook them, so you want them to be relatively dry. Sometimes I let the greens sit all night in the colander to drain. You can even roll the greens in a flour sack towel to absorb the extra water.

However, the greens do not need to be bone dry before you cook them. Even if they're wet, you'll just have extra green juice on the bottom of the pot after you cook them. My sister, Patricia, loves to drink this juice. If that's a bit too weird for you, after you remove the greens from the pot, let the extra juice simmer and thicken. Pour the thickened juice over the vegetables, and serve.

These leafy green vegetables really cook down to nothing. If you start with two big bags of spinach, you'll end up with just a couple of cups of cooked spinach.

The Greeks add a squeeze of fresh lemon juice on the greens just before eating them. Maybe the acid from the lemon helps the body absorb the vitamins. They've been doing this for thousands of years, so there must be something to it.

> 2 bags spinach or any green leafy vegetable
> 4 tablespoons olive oil, or enough oil to barely coat the bottom of a large pot
> 6 garlic cloves, lightly crushed (not too crushed or else the small bits will burn)
> Kosher salt
> Ground black pepper

On a medium-high flame, heat the pot with the olive oil; add the garlic. As soon as the garlic starts to turn golden brown, add ⅓ of the greens. Sprinkle with salt and pepper. Add the second batch, and sprinkle with more salt and pepper. You're adding the salt and pepper in between each batch so it doesn't all get concentrated in one layer of the vegetables.

Using your tongs, turn the greens. Lift the bottom layer of greens up, allowing the top layers to end up on the bottom.

Cook until wilted. Remove the cooked greens from the pot, and allow any remaining juice to evaporate and concentrate by continuing to simmer the liquid. Pour the concentrated juice over the greens.

Cauliflower with Garlic

You may have seen other recipes that call for the cauliflower to be blanched first. Blanching is just a quick boil in salted water for a minute or two. I never bother because it's just one more pot to wash. By putting the cover on the pan, you can steam the cauliflower until it's partially or even almost completely cooked. Then remove the lid for the florets to brown, and absorb the flavor of the garlic.

1 head cauliflower
5–10 garlic cloves
Olive oil (approximately 4 tablespoons)
Coarse kosher salt, to taste
Black pepper, to taste

With a sharp knife, split the sections of the cauliflower into florets. Put the florets into a sieve, and rinse briefly with cold water. Toss the florets to shake off the excess water. Set aside.

Pour the olive oil into the bottom of a large cast-iron pan, non-stick frying pan, or other large sauté pan. Make sure you have a lid that fits the pan, more or less. A lid that is a bit too small or a bit too big will suffice. Heat the oil on a medium flame. Add the garlic. The garlic will start to turn golden brown in a just a few minutes.

When the garlic begins to turn golden brown, *carefully* add the cauliflower. They are still damp from the rinsing, so the oil will splatter. You can avoid getting spattered by aiming the sieve with the cauliflower away from you. Tilt the sieve, and gently ease the cauliflower into the pan by shaking the sieve from side to side. Do it quickly and all at once because if you only get a few of the florets into the pan, it will start sputtering and splattering oil. You won't be able to get near the pan to add the rest of the cauliflower.

Sprinkle the cauliflower with salt and pepper. Put the lid on the pan for a few minutes to steam the cauliflower. Half the time, I don't bother with the lid. It's just one more thing to wash. If you skip the lid part, you'll need to sauté the cauliflower a bit longer, at a lower temperature.

After a minute, remove the lid. Start shaking the pan to turn the cauliflower. If your kitchen techniques are still elementary, use a wooden spoon to turn the florets.

The cauliflower is done when the florets are golden brown on 2 or 3 sides, after approximately 10 minutes. They will brown more quickly in a cast-iron frying pan or in a stainless steel sauté pan. Nonstick pans do not brown foods very well because they do not conduct heat as well.

Brussels Sprouts, Shallots (or Onions), and Garlic

This recipe is a variation of the cauliflower recipe. You can use it for any round vegetable; brussels sprouts and cauliflower are just an example of the possibilities.

Shallots are a pain to clean. You can use small onions instead.

As a variation of the cauliflower recipe, everything is the same except that the brussels sprouts need to cook longer. Do this by keeping the lid on longer to steam them until they're cooked almost all the way through. You could give the sprouts a quick boil before you sauté them, but that just makes one more pot to wash.

You can skip the shallots or onion, and just make this dish with brussels sprouts and garlic. It's equally as delicious.

2 small containers brussels sprouts (approximately 1 pound)
10–20 shallots or small onions, peeled
5–10 garlic cloves, peeled, whole
Olive oil (approximately 4 tablespoons)
Coarse kosher salt, to taste
Black pepper, to taste

With a sharp paring knife, clean the brussels sprouts by trimming the outer leaves and the base of the stem. Cut an *X* or a cross into the base, approximately ¼ inch deep. This helps the thicker stem cook faster; otherwise, the stem would be raw, and the leaves would be overcooked. Put into a sieve. Rinse briefly with cold water. Shake off the excess water. Set aside.

Pour the olive oil into the bottom of a large cast-iron pan or another large sauté pan with a lid. You'll want at least ⅛ or ¼ inch of oil in the bottom of the pan. If you are fatphobic, you can use a nonstick pan and use less oil, but it just won't taste the same. You need just a bit more oil for brussels sprouts than for cauliflower since they will be cooking longer.

Heat the oil on a medium flame. Add the garlic and onions. I tend to keep the garlic whole for brussels sprouts. If you mash the garlic more vigorously, the little bits will burn and turn bitter long before the brussels sprouts are cooked.

When the garlic and onions just begin to turn golden brown, *carefully* add the brussels sprouts. Just as with the cauliflower, they will still be damp and will splatter hot oil when you add them to the pan. To avoid this, tilt the sieve away from you, over the pan's edge closest to you. Gently ease the brussels sprouts into the pan by shaking the sieve from side to side. Do it quickly and all at once. You want a bit of moisture in the pan to help the vegetable steam. It shortens the cooking time.

Let the brussels sprouts brown for a few minutes, shaking the pan every so often. Sprinkle with salt and pepper to taste. Put the lid on for approximately 10 minutes to steam the brussels sprouts. If there is not much water adherent to the vegetables, you may need to add water, ¼ cup at a time. You'll need some moisture in the pan; otherwise, the brussels sprouts will stick and burn.

After the brussels sprouts have steamed and have turned bright green, remove the lid. Continue to sauté the brussels sprouts until they are golden brown. Taste one first to make sure it's done. Raw brussels sprouts are bitter. If they're still raw, put the lid back on and steam them a bit longer. This is really the way to cook them: lid on, lid off, lid on, lid off. Keep checking them. See how they look. Let them steam for a few minutes, and then, take off the top and let them brown. If they are getting brown too quickly but are still raw on the inside, lower the heat and put the lid back on. You cannot just put the lid on for 10 minutes, forget about them, and then take the lid off to let them brown. You need to check on them every few minutes. Depending on how high your flame is, how much oil you use, what kind of pan you're using, and how fresh the Brussels sprouts are, the cooking time will differ. Plus, you have a bit of leeway with the recipe. If you're fatphobic, use just a skim of oil in the pan, but you must steam the brussels sprouts for a longer period of time. You'll need to add more cooking water at some point. You could use broth instead, which will add a nice flavor.

If you love your brussels sprouts with crispy brown, caramelized outer leaves, you'll need to use more oil but steam it for a shorter period of time. You'll figure it out.

Broccoli with Garlic and Bread Crumb Topping

Broccoli really cannot be made the same way as the cauliflower or brussels sprouts because broccoli absorbs too much oil. This is a way to make broccoli tasty, so even the kids will like it.

1 bunch broccoli
4 garlic cloves, finely minced or pressed through a garlic
     press
4 tablespoons olive oil
½ cup bread crumbs
½ cup grated Parmesan cheese
¼ teaspoon black pepper

Clean the broccoli by cutting the florets off with a sharp paring knife. The stems are actually tasty and can also be used, but you need to remove the tough skin. Cut off the dried-out bottom of the main stem until you get to the part that looks fresh and moist. Peel off the tough outer layer of skin; it will come right off. You could actually set the stems aside and chop them into a salad. The stems have a crunchy, fresh flavor, almost like water chestnuts.

Rinse the broccoli florets (and stems if you're using them) in a sieve. Shake to remove excess water. Either steam the broccoli in a saucepot with ½ inch water on the bottom, or microwave them with a loose fitting lid until they turn bright green. This usually takes just a couple of minutes. Do not overcook them because you'll be baking the broccoli before serving.

Be careful when you remove the broccoli from the microwave. They will be very hot. Condensed steam will drip off the top; you can get a nasty burn that way. Make sure there are no pets or children under foot either.

Combine the olive oil, bread crumbs, grated cheese, and black pepper in a small bowl. It will have the consistency of wet sand. Turn the florets into a baking pan. Sprinkle the bread crumb mixture over the broccoli. Bake until lightly browned on top.

Roasted Asparagus with Lemon

This is really easy.

1 bunch asparagus
1–2 tablespoons olive oil
½ lemon, sliced into very thin round slices
Kosher or other large-grain salt, to taste
Black pepper, to taste

Give the asparagus a quick rinse. Snap off the tough stems at the end of each asparagus stalk. Then, snap each stalk into 3 pieces. Each piece will end up being approximately 3 or 4 inches long. Break the spear end into longer pieces and the stalk end into shorter pieces. The spears cook faster than the stems; leave them a little longer in length.

Place all of your asparagus and the thinly sliced lemon into a baking pan. Pour your olive oil over the asparagus and lemon slices. Sprinkle with kosher salt and ground black pepper. Toss.

Roast at 350 degrees for 10 to 15 minutes, turning once or twice.

Sautéed Fennel, Celery, and Onions

Some find fennel to be an unusual flavor, but cooking it makes the flavor less intense. Plus, by cooking it with celery and onion, the anise flavor of the fennel is complemented. Shallots are less intense than onions and are perfect for this dish. However, shallots are a lot of trouble to clean, and they're expensive. Onions are a perfectly acceptable alternative.

To clean the fennel, you'll need to cut off the green stems on top. You can save the stems and feathery fronds to make a soup. But for this recipe, you'll just be using the bulbs. At the base of the bulb, you'll see a tough white core in the stem. By cutting the bulb into quarters, you'll be able to remove the core without wasting any of the bulb.

Slice the bulb into thin ribbons, cutting against the grain. The thinner the slice, the faster it cooks. Try to make the size of the slices of the fennel match the size of the slices of onion and celery, so everything cooks evenly.

This recipe calls for water or broth, which helps steam the vegetables. You don't need to do this, but you'll use less oil if you use a bit of cooking liquid.

You could do this recipe with other vegetables: peppers, celery, and onions; zucchini, celery, and onions; or any combination of these. Remember, green peppers take longer to cook than other vegetables. Zucchini, on the other hand, cook quickly and give off a lot of liquid. You'll figure it out.

2 heads fennel, washed and sliced into thin slivers against the grain
½ head celery, washed and sliced on the diagonal
3 onions, sliced
½ cup water or chicken broth
2 tablespoons olive oil
Salt
Pepper

In a large sauté or frying pan, heat the oil. Add the onions first, and let cook for 2 or 3 minutes; then, add the fennel. These take longer to cook, so you want to give them a head start. Add the celery. Sprinkle with salt and pepper. If you put the lid on the pan, the vegetables will steam, and you'll need less olive oil. As they cook, see how much liquid they give off. Add some water or broth if the vegetables are beginning to stick to the bottom of the pan. Likewise, if the edges of the vegetables are burning while the centers are still raw, you need to add some liquid or a bit more oil.

Sauté until the vegetables are wilted but not mushy.

Giambotta and Caponata

Giambotta is a dish of vegetables sautéed in olive oil. It always starts with garlic and onions and ends with tomatoes. In between, you can use zucchini, eggplant, or peppers. You could mix and match, or you could use all three together, but I don't recommend it. The cooking times of zucchini, peppers, and eggplant are too different. If you're not an experienced cook, it will make you crazy. The eggplant will still be raw as the zucchini turns into mush. Plus, using eggplant, zucchini, and peppers all together are just too many flavors. It won't taste very good.

The recipe for giambotta listed here will use peppers. Red peppers cook faster than green peppers. That means you would let the onions cook longer before adding the red peppers. If you use green peppers, add them to the onions early. You would only need to let the onions cook a minute or two before adding the green peppers.

If you decide to use zucchini, you must slice and then salt the zucchini ahead of time. Let the salted zucchini stand in a sieve. When they start giving off liquid, remove the zucchini one handful at a time and squeeze out the excess water. The longer they sit, the more water can be squeezed out. Since the zucchini are salted, do not add much more salt during cooking.

If you're making caponata, you'll be slicing the eggplant ahead of time. Salt the sliced eggplant, and let them sit in a colander for an hour or so. This seems to reduce the bitterness and softens the eggplant. Squeeze out the excess water before cooking. Capers and vinegar are used to flavor the caponata. Do not add salt until the very end, after you taste the vegetables. The capers and olives are salty. The eggplant is salted before you cook it. True, you squeeze out the extra water from the eggplant and lose some of the salt that way, but it still retains some. Just before serving, taste the vegetables for seasoning. It probably won't need any more salt.

Giambotta	Caponata
3 garlic cloves, smashed	3 garlic cloves, smashed
3 large onions, sliced	2 large onions, sliced
3 red bell peppers, sliced	1 eggplant, peeled and
1 can plum tomatoes	sliced
4 tablespoons olive oil	1 can plum tomatoes
5–6 leaves of fresh, or 1	4 tablespoons olive oil
tablespoon dried, basil	2 tablespoons capers
½ cup fresh, or 2 table-	½ cup olives (any color)
spoons dried, parsley	¼ cup fresh basil
Salt	Black pepper
Black pepper	Splash of red wine vinegar

If you're making caponata, salt the sliced eggplant. Set the eggplant aside in a sieve to drain for an hour or more. Squeeze out any excess water, a handful of eggplant at a time.

Add the olive oil to a sauté pan. Heat the pan, and add the cloves of garlic. When you hear the garlic sizzle, add the onions. When the edges of the onions begin to turn translucent, add the red peppers or the eggplant.

If you're making giambotta, add a sprinkle of salt. You do not need to do this for caponata.

Season the vegetables with ground black pepper. Add your basil and parsley. Add the capers and olives if you're making caponata. Let cook for 10 minutes until the vegetables are tender but not mushy. Add the splash of vinegar to the caponata.

Taste and adjust the seasonings.

Winter Squash: Acorn and Butternut

Since I tend to cook for a couple of days at a time, I usually make two or three, depending on the size of the squash. Stay away from the very large ones. They are simply too hard to handle. How many you decide to cook also depends on your baking pans. The squash will be cut in half and then laid cut side down in the pan. If you don't have a large baking pan, only make what can fit in the pan you own.

The hardest part is splitting the squash open. With the cleaver you bought in Chinatown, find a stable way to sit the squash on one end. If your chopping board isn't stable, put a dishtowel under the board. The board won't slip around that way. Carefully, make your first cut in the squash by cleaving it near the top. The cleaver will probably stick in the squash. Good! That's what you want. Then, lifting the cleaver with the blade stuck in the squash, pound the whole thing down. This will force your blade through the squash. Trying to split the squash into two even pieces is an art.

If you do not own a cleaver, do not attempt this recipe. It's not worth a trip to the emergency room. Even if you have a very sharp, large chef's knife, you won't be able to cut through the squash. You need a cleaver for the job.

> 2 acorn squash
> 2 butternut squash
> Water, to simmer the squash in the pan
> Brown sugar, dark brown is preferable
> Cinnamon or pumpkin pie spice

Cut the squash in half, lengthwise, as explained above. With a metal spoon, scoop out the seeds and discard. Lay the squash, cut side down, in a large baking pan. Add water until it comes ½ inch up the side of the squash.

Bake in 350-degree oven for approximately 1 hour, or until the squash has some give to it when pressed. Check the squash 30 minutes into the baking, and add more water if all the water has evaporated. You don't need a lot of water in the bottom of the pan. You'll need just enough to make sure the squash don't stick to the bottom of the pan. If you add too much water, you risk splashing yourself with boiling hot water when you take the pan out of oven.

When the squash are almost done, they'll have some give when pressed, but won't be mushy. Take the pan out of the oven, and turn each squash over so the cut side is now facing up. Sprinkle each squash with brown sugar and cinnamon or pumpkin pie spice. Some people add a pat of butter, but it really isn't necessary. Return to the oven for another 5 to 10 minutes. The squash are ready when the sugar is melted.

If you don't own a large baking pan, another way to cook these is by wrapping them in aluminum foil. After you have scooped out the seeds, wrap each half of squash separately in foil. Make sure the folded portion of the foil is on top, facing up. If the folded edge is on the bottom, when you bake it, juice from the squash might leak out and make a mess in your oven. When the squash are cooked, open the foil, and sprinkle the top with the brown sugar and cinnamon. Rewrap the squash and stick it in the oven for a few more minutes so the sugar melts.

Soups

You probably aren't going to be cooking soups during the summer, but during the winter, a hearty soup can be a satisfying meal. Best of all, most soups freeze well, so you can make a big pot, and freeze the leftovers for dinner another night.

Spinach and Beans

This is a true fifteen-minute meal: fast, easy, inexpensive, and delicious.

Beans alone are not a complete protein, which means they are missing a few amino acids for human needs. If you add a grain to a bean dish, you'll have a complete protein. You could have brown rice or barley on the side or a slice of whole wheat bread. You could make the spinach and beans a bit soupier by adding water or stock and do as the French and the Italians do: Put a piece of dried-out old French or Italian bread on the bottom of the bowl. Pour the soup on top, and let it soak into the bread.

Using fennel in this dish is optional. Though it's very healthy, it may be an unusual flavor for some people, especially the first time they taste it. Most people who try this dish love it. There are a few people who hate it, but they're in the minority.

The dish is much tastier if you use fresh spinach instead of frozen spinach. But if your time is tight, use the frozen. It's still delicious.

There have been times when I didn't have frozen spinach in the house. You could substitute frozen kale or mustard greens. My grandmother used to make this dish with escarole, which is a very bitter green. The problem is that I've never seen packages of frozen escarole in the supermarket, and escarole is a pain in the neck to clean. It's one of those vegetables that must be very good for you because it starts out so dirty.

> 1 19-oz. can cannellini (white kidney) beans
> 2 packages frozen spinach
> 2 tablespoons olive oil
> 3–5 garlic cloves, whole or crushed
> 1 bay leaf (optional)
> 1–2 teaspoons fennel seeds (optional)
> Salt and pepper, to taste

Begin heating the oil in a medium saucepot, large skillet, or a large sauté pan. The amount of oil will depend on the diameter of the pot. You'll need less oil for a pot with a smaller diameter. You want ⅛ to ¼ inch oil on the bottom of the pot. Add the garlic. When the garlic just begins to turn golden, add the can of beans, juice and all. If you're adding a bay leaf, it goes in the pot now. Slowly simmer for 5 to 10 minutes.

Gently place the 2 packages of frozen spinach into the pot, without splashing yourself with hot oil. Add the fennel seeds if you are using them. Cover the pot with a lid, and let simmer until the spinach is defrosted, stirring occasionally.

Add ground black pepper to taste. It rarely ever needs more salt since the canned beans are already salted. If you're on a budget, by all means, make a pot of dried beans and freeze the extra.

Split Pea Soup

The ingredients of this soup, the split peas and the vegetables, cost around four dollars. You'll get eighteen cups of soup. That's twenty-two cents per cup of soup. What a bargain!

Our nutritionist at Boriken, who is the picture of good health and vitality, has a trick to make this soup even healthier. She buys the whole dried green peas. She doesn't buy the split peas. Then, she soaks the dried peas in water for a day or two. You'll need to change the water a couple of times. She checks the peas for germination. Just when she sees the little sprouts sticking out of the peas, she cooks the peas as she would regular split pea soup. She says the germination does something to the enzymes in the peas, which makes the nutrients more available to be absorbed by our digestive system.

    3 tablespoons olive oil
    2 carrots, chopped
    2 ribs celery, chopped
    2 onions, chopped
    2 garlic cloves, smashed
    1 leftover ham bone or 2 oz. bacon, minced (optional)
    1 bag dried split peas, rinsed
    Salt and pepper, to taste

Pour the olive oil in the bottom of a large soup pot, and turn the heat to medium. If you're using bacon, put the bacon in first to begin browning. Stir often to make sure the bacon doesn't stick to the bottom. When the bacon has begun to turn brown around the edges, add the garlic, celery, carrots, and onions. Sprinkle the vegetables with a bit of salt. This helps speed the cooking process and helps the vegetables to *sweat*, which means they start giving off their water. You can put the lid on the pot for a few minutes to speed up the cooking. When the onions start to become translucent around the edges, add 6 cups of water. You can heat the water in a separate pot while the vegetables are browning in order to save some preparation time.

When the water comes to a boil, add the dried peas. Lower the heat. If you're adding a ham bone, put it in the pot now. Cover the pot, and let simmer 2 hours. The cooking time will depend on the age of the peas and how high your flame is. Stir the pot every so often to make sure the peas are not sticking on the bottom.

Salt and pepper, to taste.

Cabbage Soup

Does anyone remember that seven-day diet where you ate vegetables the first day, fruit the next day, bananas and milk another day, and so on? One of the secrets to that diet was a soup that has had a variety of names: cabbage soup, miracle soup, or my favorite name, "poop soup." One of the many versions of this soup on the Internet calls for bouillon cubes for extra flavor. I don't recommend it. Bouillon cubes have an artificial taste and are way too salty. They contain too many artificial ingredients. This soup is flavorful, so you really don't need to use bouillon cubes.

If you're feeling ambitious and want to make the soup special, use homemade broth. For hundreds, if not thousands of years, broth has been used for health. Beef broth, made from beef bones, is very easy and very inexpensive. The same goes for chicken stock. Economize. Save the bones from takeout roasted chicken in a big baggie in the freezer. When you've saved up enough bones, stick them in a big pot of water with a couple of cloves of garlic, some parsley, and a couple of onions and carrots. Simmer slowly, and you'll have a beautiful broth in no time. Do the same for beef stock. Save your bones from steak dinners. Buy inexpensive beef bones from the butcher. Economize and eat healthy, both at the same time. If you add a bit of acid to the simmering water as you cook the broth, calcium from the bones is dissolved into the broth. It's a delicious and healthy way to "eat" some extra calcium.

This soup is so flavorful, though, that you really don't need to use chicken or beef broth. Water will be just fine.

You should always have some of this cabbage soup on hand in the freezer. During the winter, have a bowl of this soup before dinner instead of a salad. You could make this soup a meal by adding beans and pasta. One four-cup container of this soup with a can of cannellini beans and a handful of pasta can be a good winter meal for two hungry people. This soup is a bit low in fat, so you may find you want to eat again two or three hours later. If you add a dollop of olive oil and some grated Parmesan cheese, the soup will hold you longer. If money is no object, buy a small bottle of really good olive oil. It will add a tremendous flavor. Plus, you need some oil in your meal in order to absorb the fat-soluble vitamins from the vegetables.

Adding pasta and beans to the soup will create what the Italians call minestrone. Do not add a pound of pasta. Just a handful or two of pasta will do the trick. You cannot cook the pasta in the soup. You must boil it separately. Pasta needs a lot of water, at a rolling boil, in order to cook properly. Do not overcook the pasta; cook it al dente. The literal translation of al dente is, "to the tooth," which means the pasta has a bite to it. When added to the soup, the pasta will absorb liquid from the soup. The pasta will soften up considerably, so make sure you undercook the pasta. Keep the pasta and soup separate, and then add a handful of pasta to the bowls as you serve the soup. If you end up with leftover soup and pasta, do not mix them together; otherwise, the pasta will become very mushy. Unless you don't mind mushy pasta, store the soup and the pasta separately.

    1 bag carrots, chopped
    1 whole celery, chopped
    1 bag onions, chopped
    1 head cabbage, chopped
    1–2 large cans whole plum tomatoes
    4–8 garlic cloves, smashed
    Salt and pepper, to taste
    2 tablespoons dried, or ½ cup fresh, basil
    1 tablespoon dried oregano
    1 tablespoon dried, or ½ cup fresh, parsley
    1 tablespoon dried savory (optional)
    Chicken or beef broth to cover all the vegetables

or

Water to cover all the vegetables

Find your biggest pot. You may need your 2 biggest pots because this recipe will make a lot of soup. Bring a quart of water to boil as you prepare the vegetables. You'll need to add more water as you go along, but start with one quart, more or less.

Add the smashed garlic. Then, add the vegetables in this order as you chop them: first, the onions; then, the carrots; then, the celery. You don't need to have everything chopped ahead of time. You can chop as you go. Try to cut the vegetables into bite-size pieces. The onions take the longest to cook, so they go into the boiling water first, and so on.

Season your soup with the salt, pepper, and herbs. The cabbage goes in next to last. Cabbage cooks relatively quickly, 10 minutes or so. When the cabbage looks like it's almost done (it becomes soft and translucent), add the can(s) of tomatoes. Let it simmer for another 10 minutes.

This recipe makes a big pot of soup. Freeze the soup in 4-cup and 8-cup containers.

Beans

If you're seriously on a budget, you should know how to cook dried beans. It's so much cheaper to make your own beans than to buy canned. You need to leave yourself some time to soak the beans, and there are variations on how to do this. Some people soak them overnight. Others do a quick boil, let them cool, and then resume cooking after the water has cooled from the first boil. You could use a pressure cooker. If you own and use a pressure cooker, you don't need to read these recipes. You know more than I do about cooking beans.

1 bag dried beans, rinsed
6 cups boiling water (generally 3 parts water to 1 part bean)
4 garlic cloves, whole (optional)

1 bay leaf (optional)
Salt, to taste

Bring the water to a boil. Drop in your beans, and rapidly bring back to a boil. Let the beans boil for 2 minutes. Remove the pot from the heat, cover with a lid, and let rest for 1 hour. Add your garlic and bay leaf. Bring the pot back to a simmer, uncovered or partially covered, for 2 hours. You'll need to add more cooking water as you go along. When the beans are almost done, add salt. Do not add the salt too soon, or else the beans will become tough. When the beans taste smooth, they are done.

Alternately, soak your dried beans overnight in plenty of water. In the morning, pour off the soaking liquid. Add fresh water to cover the beans, and your garlic and bay leaf. The water should cover the beans with an extra 2 or 3 inches to spare. Bring the water to a boil, and then reduce the flame, so the beans simmer. You can leave the pot covered or uncovered. If you leave the pot uncovered, be sure to make sure the cooking liquid does not boil off. If you cover the pot, leave the flame as low as possible so the water does not boil over and make a mess on your stove. The beans will take approximately 2 hours with this technique. Salt the beans when they're done (you'll be able to tell by tasting one.)

This will give you a lot of beans. Freeze the extra in 2-cup and 4-cup containers. Add the beans to salads or soups.

Variations

You could make a pureed soup by sautéing celery and onion in a bit of olive oil. Add some cooked beans and broth or water. Puree the beans and vegetables in the blender. The soup will be a smooth and creamy French bean soup.

You could also make a big batch of black bean soup. Make your beans as outlined above. Sauté chopped carrots, onions, and celery with a clove or two of garlic. Add your black beans and a package of frozen corn. This is another hearty winter meal.

Lentil, Tomato, and Barley Soup

Lentils are really very good for you. They are high in iron, so if you have iron-deficiency anemia, eat lentils a couple times a week. These little legumes also get your colon moving. If you suffer from constipation, this is the meal for you!

You can make the lentils, with or without the tomatoes, ahead of time and freeze the soup in serving-size containers. You won't be able to freeze the soup with the barley added for two reasons. First of all, barley does not freeze well. Secondly, if you store the barley with the lentils, the barley will absorb all of the liquid from the lentils. The soup becomes thick, and the barley becomes mushy.

This recipe calls for canned plum tomatoes. You can use leftover tomato sauce instead. When you make tomato sauce, there is always some leftover. Freeze the leftover tomato sauce, a cup here and a cup there. Defrost and use in place of the canned plum tomatoes. You could use a jar of prepared tomato sauce instead of canned tomatoes if you want. Experiment and make the recipe your own.

The recipe here is a simplified version of the traditional recipe. My mom would open the cans of tomatoes and cook them in a separate pot with two cloves of garlic and some fresh basil. That's one more step and one more pot to wash. The soup does end up being tastier by doing it her way, but not tasty enough to be worth an extra dirty pot.

The proportion of lentils to tomatoes to barley is not set in stone. If you're watching your carbohydrates, use less barley. If you don't have two cans of tomatoes, use just one. If you like vegetables in your soup, use more onions, carrots, and celery. If you hate onions, use less. You get the idea.

Wild rice, which is not that expensive, is also good in this dish. Use the wild rice in place of the barley. Since wild rice is a more complex carbohydrate than barley, it's probably better to use than the barley. Wild rice is a better choice if you want to eat high-glycemic-index carbohydrates.

1 bag lentils
2 large, or 3 small, onions, chopped
2–3 carrots, chopped
2–3 celery ribs, chopped
2 garlic cloves, lightly crushed
4 tablespoons olive oil
1 bay leaf
½ cup fresh, or 2 tablespoons dried, parsley
½ cup fresh, or 1 tablespoon dried, basil
⅔ cup barley
6 cups water plus 1 to 2 additional cups of water for the
    barley
1–2 cans plum tomatoes
Salt, to taste
Black pepper, to taste

Over medium heat, pour the olive oil into a large pot. There should be just enough olive oil to coat the bottom of the pan. Add the crushed garlic. When the garlic begins to sizzle, add the chopped onions, celery, and carrot. Sprinkle with a bit of salt and pepper. The salt helps the vegetables to sweat, which means they give off some liquid, and cook faster. Cook the vegetables for 10 minutes, or until they just begin to soften. Putting the lid on the pot will help the vegetables cook faster, if you're in a hurry.

Meanwhile, open the bag of lentils. You should go through the lentils to look for little stones or bits of dirt. My mom would pour the lentils onto a big board and pick through each lentil. I don't bother because I haven't found a stone in years. Instead, I slowly pour the lentils from the bag into a fine-mesh sieve. As I pour, I keep a lookout for small objects that don't belong. Then, rinse the lentils right in the sieve.

When the onions are slightly translucent, you're ready to add the water and lentils. Do so carefully. The lentils will have stuck together in the sieve, so you'll need to loosen them up with a wooden spoon or by hand. Add the bay leaf. Cover. Bring to a boil; then, lower the heat so the soup is just at a simmer. Stir every so often to make sure the lentils are not sticking to the bottom of the pot.

Cook for 1 to 2 hours, until the lentils are soft but not falling apart. Add the cans of tomatoes, season with the parsley and basil, and then cook for an additional 10 to 20 minutes.

Just after you add the tomatoes, bring 1 to 2 cups of salted water to boil in a separate pot for the barley. When the water is at a boil, add the barley, and cook until it's a bit under-cooked, stirring every so often. It will absorb liquid from the lentils and get softer.

Combine the barley with the lentil-tomato soup just before you're ready to serve dinner. Don't mix the whole pot of barley with the whole pot of lentil-tomato soup. The barley will absorb all of the liquid from the soup, so keep them separate. Ladle the soup into individual serving bowls, and then add a couple of heaping tablespoons of the barley to each individual bowl.

You'll have plenty of leftover lentil soup. Freeze the extra, but remember, don't freeze the barley with the lentils, or else the barley will absorb all of the liquid from the lentils and become mushy.

Salads and Salad Dressings

A typical salad in any Mediterranean country is simply salad greens with olive oil and vinegar, sprinkled with salt and pepper. Any kind of vinegar will do, but red wine vinegar is traditional. Think about it! There are grapes grown in numerous Mediterranean countries—Portugal, Spain, France, Italy, and Greece. Every grandfather made wine in the basement, and he set aside a barrel to make wine vinegar to use on salads in the coming year. I still have a few bottles I inherited from various relatives through the years. The stuff will put hair on your chest.

You need to use vinegar sparingly. The ratio should be three parts oil to one part vinegar. Folklore says to pour the oil on the salad first, so the vinegar has something to hold onto. What makes more sense to me is that if you pour the vinegar first, the oil will not stick to the greens because they are wet. However, Rachael Ray puts the vinegar first. She says the vinegar will not stick to the greens if you put the oil first. Do it whichever way you want: oil first or vinegar first.

So after your salad is washed and dried, dress it with your olive oil and vinegar. Sprinkle it with coarse salt and ground pepper, toss, and you're done. If one starts with fresh, tasty greens, a salad doesn't need anything more than good olive oil, decent vinegar, salt, and pepper. If you do not like red wine vinegar, use balsamic vinegar.

Fennel Salad

You need to slice the fennel into fairly thin slices. If you don't have a sharp knife, do not try to prepare this salad. People cut themselves when they try to force dull knives through food.

> 1–2 heads fennel
> Juice of ½ a lemon
> Kosher salt
> Black pepper

Remove the stems (tops) of the fennel, which are tough. Slice the head of fennel in half, from the top down through the bulb. The bottom, center of the bulb has a hard core. You can either remove the core, or slice it into the salad. Taste it. If it's not too tough and bitter, use it. Fennel is too expensive to waste. After you separate the stalks of fennel from the core, rinse off any dirt. Drain.

Slice the fennel stalks, across the grain, into very thin slices. Toss with olive oil and the lemon juice. Sprinkle with salt and pepper to taste. Let the salad sit a few minutes before serving, so the lemon juice softens the fennel slices.

Parsley and Carrot Salad with Lemon Juice and Olive Oil

This one salad is off-the-charts full of antioxidants. You may not think the anchovies are necessary, but the lemon really cuts the saltiness and fishiness. The anchovies add flavor, as well as omega-3 fatty acids. This recipe is adapted from a salad Jacques Pépin prepared on his PBS cooking show. You may think Food Network is the only place to see a cooking show on TV. Actually, there is a PBS station in the Northeast (WLIW Create) with cooking and home improvement shows all day long. Best of all, there are no commercials.

The longest part of this salad is washing the parsley. You could pick off each leaf individually, which is a long and tedious process. Don't bother. Just wash the bunch of parsley, set it aside to drain, wrap it in a flour sack towel to blot off the extra moisture, and then chop.

1 bunch parsley, washed
3–4 carrots, depending on their size
Juice of 1 lemon
4–8 tablespoons olive oil
Kosher salt
Black pepper
1 garlic clove, smashed
3–4 anchovies (optional)

Wash the parsley; set it to drain in a colander. Wash the carrots and grate using the side of the grater with the ⅜-inch-wide holes. Don't use the small holes, which are for grating cheese. Don't use the biggest holes, which are for making ribbons of carrots or cucumber.

Puree the lemon juice, olive oil, salt, pepper, and anchovies together in a small mini-prep, a bullet, or your blender. Since you'll have little chunks of garlic left in the dressing, pass the dressing through a small fine-mesh sieve.

The parsley can be a bit tough, especially if the sprouts are mature and not young. Letting the dressed salad sit in the refrigerator for 1 hour will soften them up. Leftovers of this salad keep well. You'll have leftovers because you cannot eat a lot of this salad. The parsley gets to you after a while.

Balsamic Vinegar

Decent balsamic vinegar is really very expensive. The inexpensive balsamic vinegar you can get in any supermarket is not very tasty and has a hard acidic edge to it. If you marinate the vinegar with dried fruits, it takes an inexpensive bottle of balsamic and turns it into something far more enjoyable. This recipe calls for dried figs. You can try different combinations: figs, raisins, or dried cherries. You could try adding a couple tablespoons of brown sugar. Since molasses is so good for you, I've tried adding a couple of tablespoons, but it adds a bitter edge to the vinegar. It just isn't right for a salad. You could add some lemon peel, but the oils in the peel will go rancid, so you'll have to refrigerate the prepared vinegar and use it within a couple of weeks.

1 bottle inexpensive balsamic vinegar
½ package dried figs
2 tablespoons brown sugar (optional)

Empty the contents of the vinegar bottle into a saucepan. Add the brown sugar, and heat over a low flame until the sugar dissolves. Remove from the heat. Break the figs in half and place into the vinegar. Cool. Refrigerate.

Store the vinegar and figs, refrigerated, in a glass bottle. You'll never get the vinegar and figs back into the original vinegar bottle. Try to save some wide-mouthed jars, like the ones that wheat germ comes in. You'll need a wide-mouthed jar in order to fish out the figs.

Do not waste those figs marinating in the vinegar. Use the figs on your salad too! A couple of the figs are delicious chopped in a salad, especially the *tuna over salad with balsamic vinegar* recipe.

Tuna over Salad with Balsamic Vinegar

This is really easy. It takes five minutes from start to finish.

To make this salad into a more satisfying meal, add a chopped baked potato or croutons.

2 cans chunk light tuna in olive oil (1 can per person)

1 head radicchio (or ½ head, depending on how large the
head is)
1 head endive
Olive oil
Balsamic vinegar
Black pepper

This is a 5-minute meal, and I have no desire to separate the heads into individual leaves, and then, wash, spin, and dry them. Who has that kind of time? Instead, pull off the outermost leaves as those leaves are the ones most likely to be dirty. Then, rinse the outside of the heads and pat them dry. If you worry about germs, go ahead and wash them as you would any other lettuce or leafy vegetable. Chop.

Place the chopped radicchio and endive into a bowl. Put the 2 cans of tuna, including the oil, over the chopped radicchio and endive. The oil from the canned tuna is never enough for this salad—you'll need a little extra. Pour a bit more olive oil over the salad. Pour balsamic vinegar over the salad to taste. Add ground black pepper to taste. Mix. Top with croutons, if you have any, for crunch, or a cubed baked potato. There is enough salt in the tuna. You won't need to add any extra.

There are a number of variations on this salad:

Add a chopped red onion
Use different types of greens: spinach, mesclun, Boston or
romaine lettuce
Add chopped sun-dried tomatoes
Add a jar or can of artichoke hearts
Throw in a few black olives

Tomato Salad

If you make this salad ahead of time, the tomatoes give off quite a bit of juice. My grandmother used to make this, and the kids went crazy over it. We loved dipping bread into the juice. Since we cannot eat that much bread anymore, and since supermarket tomatoes are awful, I'll make this salad when I can get farm-fresh tomatoes at the farmer's market. Serve it on the side of steak and a baked potato because you can dip the steak and the potato into the juice.

There are no quantities listed because you need to go by feel.

Tomatoes
Olive oil
Salt
Black pepper
Basil, fresh is preferable
Oregano

Cut the tomatoes into slices. Drizzle with olive oil. Sprinkle with salt and pepper. Sprinkle with some oregano (not too much though; otherwise, it can become bitter). Add a few leaves of basil. Toss and let rest for 30 minutes.

Roasted Beet Salad

The best part of a beet is the green leafy top. I always try to buy beets with the tops still attached. Beet greens are delicious sautéed in a bit of olive oil and garlic.

As for the beets, after they are roasted, you'll need to peel the skin. Use a pair of disposable latex gloves, or paper towels; otherwise, you'll stain your hands and nails.

There are lots of different things you could do with beets roasted this way. Restaurants serve a chopped roasted beet salad over endive leaves as an appetizer. The recipe here does not call for any vinegar or lemon juice, but you could add either one if you plan to serve the roasted beets with salad greens like endive or romaine. You could sprinkle chopped roasted beets with pecans and crumbled blue cheese. Let your imagination go wild.

1 bunch beets, washed
½ red onion, cut into thin slices
1–2 tablespoons olive oil

Kosher salt

Black pepper

Remove the green leafy tops as close to the root as possible. Cut through the greens and not through the root, or else you'll lose beet juice from the cut end. Reserve the greens to sauté in olive oil and garlic.

Wash the beets to remove loose dirt. There's no need to scrub them until they're spotless; you'll be peeling the beets after they are roasted. Wrap each beet in aluminum foil. You'll need to curl the tail of the beet around. You don't want it sticking out of the foil. Do not cut off the long, thin tail either. If you do, the beet will lose a lot of juice, even though the opening you cut may be very small.

Bake for an hour, more or less, at about 350 degrees. The baking time will depend on the size of the beets and how fresh they are. For small beets, check them in 30 minutes. When you press on the wrapped beet, it should have a little give but not be mushy. Large beets can take as long as 1 to 2 hours to cook. The temperature is flexible too, especially if you're multitasking and are baking something else in the oven at a different temperature. Just cook the beets longer at a lower temperature, or shorter at a higher temperature. You could put the wrapped beets in a baking dish. If the beet juice does leek out of the foil, you won't have a mess in the oven.

There's another technique to roast beets if you don't want to wrap each one individually in foil. You could place your beets in a roasting pan and drizzle a bit of olive oil on top of each one. Add ⅛ inch water to the roasting pan. The water prevents burning, and it helps the beets cook faster by steaming them. Cover the pan tightly with foil, and bake in the oven at 350 degrees for an hour or so.

When the beets are cooked, remove them from the oven. Let cool. Peel and slice. Add the thinly sliced red onion. Pour the olive oil over the salad. Sprinkle with salt and ground black pepper to taste. Toss. Serve at room temperature or chilled.

Breakfast Shake

There are some tricks that will make it quick and easy to make a breakfast shake in the morning.

If you're using frozen fruit, defrost it the night before. Pour out the amount of fruit into a bowl or glass. Put it in the refrigerator overnight. The fruit will be defrosted, but still cold, by the next morning.

If you know the morning will be hectic, prepare the ingredients the night before. Measure the green vegetable powder, protein powder, and peanut butter into one container. Have the frozen fruit defrosting in the refrigerator. In the morning, throw everything in the blender with a cup of milk. Your shake can be ready in a minute.

Although blueberries are a powerhouse fruit, it's probably a good idea to mix it up with peaches, cherries, apples, or whatever strikes your fancy. Mangos can be a bit too stringy for a shake, but you can find frozen mangos in your supermarket. Bananas will make the shake too thick, but you can use one if you like.

You can alternate between different nut butters as well; peanut is the cheapest. The health food stores usually carry cashew butter and almond butter, but they are considerably more expensive.

I stopped using protein powder in my shakes for a little while over concerns that the protein might be hydrolyzed, which means it might not be very good for you. Ideally, the best protein powder to use is one that is cold processed. Cold processing does not denature the milk proteins. Cold-processed whey is very, very expensive when you can find it. Regular whey protein powder is probably okay. As a matter of fact, there is considerable data showing whey protein powder is actually good for you.

If you try to make a shake without extra protein from protein powder, the shake might not hold your hunger until lunchtime. I tried using yogurt instead of the protein powder, but I was still getting hungry after a couple of hours. I'm back to using protein powder. Go ahead and use protein powder if you find the shake does not hold you until lunchtime. The only flavor of protein powder to use is natural flavor. Do not buy French vanilla or chocolate. They are far too sweet. Do not buy soy protein. It has a chalky taste and is really disgusting. Do not buy off-brand protein powders. Designer Protein and Jarrow are excellent brands. There are even goat's milk protein powders you can buy over the Internet. I've tried them all, and I recommend Designer Protein Natural Flavor. It's easier to find than the other brands. Other brands, like Jarrow, will only be at health food stores whereas Designer Protein is available at GNC and other supplement stores.

If you find you're still getting hungry after a couple of hours, another trick is to increase the amount of fats in the shake. Use extra nut butter if you're getting hungry too soon before lunch. The oils in the nut butters will hold you until lunchtime. Also, tree nut butters, like almond butter, will hold you better than peanut butter, which is a legume. Even better is to add flaxseed oil, about half a tablespoon per serving, to the shake. If you use any more than half a tablespoon, it gives the shake a fishy odor, even though it doesn't have a fishy taste. Our nutritionist, Olga, doesn't believe in flaxseed oil because it turns rancid too quickly. She recommends the ground seeds, which would make the shake too thick to drink through a straw.

> 1–2 cups frozen blueberries
> 1 tablespoon (at least) peanut butter, or other nut butter
> 1 scoop fruit and vegetable extract powder (see appendix 7)
> 1 scoop protein powder
> 1 cup milk
> ½ tablespoon flaxseed oil (optional)

Always put the fruit into the blender first. If you put the powder and nut butter in first and then the fruit on top of that, you'll get a sticky mess on the bottom of the blender. I've tried all different ways. If you put the powder in last, after the milk, the powder sticks in a ring around the top of the liquid level. Learn from my mistakes. Always assemble the ingredients in exactly this sequence:

1. Fruit goes into the blender.

2. Next, add the green powder and the protein powder. Using a knife, stir the fruit around. You want the powders to sink into the fruit. You don't want the powder to stick to the glass of the blender.

3. Put the dollop of nut butter on top of the fruit. Keep it away from the glass of the blender, or else it will stick to the glass.

4. If you're using flaxseed oil, you can add it now.

5. Add your milk.

6. Blend. When you pour your shake out, if you see little round pieces of blueberries, you didn't blend it enough. Put it back, and blend it for another minute. If, after all that blending, there are still chunks of blueberries, it means the blades on your blender are dull. You need to buy a new blender.

7. If you're using blueberries, always drink your shake with a straw. Do not get pieces of blueberry on your teeth. Blueberries can stain. Brush your teeth after the shake if you can.

Do not be disturbed by the color of the blueberry shake. It will be a dark greenish-grayish-purple.

Drink.

Bon appétit.

Appendix One

Produce to Buy Organic

I f you cannot go totally organic, there's a list of vegetables you should buy organic. This list has been has been bandied around. I've seen it in magazines and on the Internet.

There are some vegetables that bugs just don't like, so the crops aren't sprayed with a lot of pesticides. There are others that have a thick skin, so the pesticides don't penetrate the skin. These are safe to buy nonorganic, like bananas and avocados. Other foods have thin skins that absorb pesticides easily, like strawberries. Green leafy vegetables, like spinach, which grow close to the ground, likewise absorb chemicals easily. Sweet fruits, like cherries, are heavily sprayed to keep bugs away. Bugs, birds, and humans love sweet fruits. Foods they say you should buy organic are:

Imported grapes (nonorganic grapes from the United States are okay)

Apples

Bell peppers

Celery

Nectarines

Peaches

Pears

Potatoes
Raspberries
Strawberries
Cherries
Carrots
Lettuce
Spinach, and other green leafy vegetables

An excellent book to look at is *To Buy or Not to Buy Organic* by Cindy Burke. Ms. Burke goes through each fruit and vegetable and tells you when you should buy organic, or when it's safe to buy nonorganic. I highly recommend this informative book.

Appendix Two

Menu Ideas

Winter Menu

	Monday	Tuesday	Wednesday	Thursday	Friday
Breakfast	Blueberry shake	2 eggs and a slice of whole wheat toast	Blueberry shake	Bowl of oatmeal and 2 eggs	Blueberry shake
Mid-morning snack	2-ounce bag of almonds and an orange	Walnuts and a cup of grapes	Zone bar or other high-protein bar	One hard-boiled egg and an orange	Cup of chicken broth
Lunch	Min-estrone with beans and pasta	Spinach and bean soup and a leftover baked sweet potato	Split pea soup	Lentil-barley soup	Leftover minestrone

	Monday	Tuesday	Wednesday	Thursday	Friday
After-noon snack	Can of V8 juice and a piece of cheese	Can of sardines on whole grain crackers	Walnuts and a banana	One left-over link of sausage and a piece of fruit	3 carrots and a handful of olives or nuts
Dinner	Lamb chops, a baked sweet potato, and a side of sautéed greens	Fish stew over wild rice with a side of a green leafy veg-etable	Pasta (one cup only) with sautéed vegetables on top, a side of cauliflower, and two links of sausage	Min-estrone with pasta and beans	Three bean stew with pasta or rice

Summer Menu

	Monday	Tuesday	Wednesday	Thursday	Friday
Breakfast	Blueberry shake	2 eggs and a slice of whole wheat toast	Blueberry shake	Bowl of oatmeal and 2 eggs	Blueberry shake
Mid-morning snack	2-ounce bag of almonds and an orange	Grapes and nuts	Guacamole with carrot sticks and sliced cucumber for dipping	More guacamole with carrot sticks and sliced cucumber for dipping	Carrot sticks and a piece of leftover chicken
Lunch	Yogurt with fruit, nuts, and granola	Can of tuna and boiled potatoes on a bed of arugula with balsamic vinegar	Can of sardines and a sliced avocado on a bed of lettuce	Leftover chicken on a bed of salad greens with olive oil and vinegar	Leftover steak and baked potato sliced and tossed into a salad
Afternoon snack	Can of V8 juice and a piece of cheese	Cashews and a peach	Piece of cheese and an apple	Nuts and some grapes	Mixed olives and fresh radishes
Dinner	Frittata with cheese and vegetables, tomato salad, and whole wheat bread	Cod fish salad with avocado	Chicken, brown rice, sautéed greens, and butternut squash	Steak, a baked potato, asparagus with lemon, and a tomato salad	Salmon, sautéed Swiss chard, ⅔ cup wild rice, and artichoke heart salad

Appendix Three

Outfit Your Kitchen

Pots and pans:
   One 9-inch or 10-inch sauté pan with a lid
   One 4-quart pot with a lid
   One 8-quart pot with a lid
   Large stockpot
   One 14-inch skillet
   One roasting pan
Wooden spoons and spatulas
Blender for making shakes in the morning
Mixing bowls in three sizes: small, medium, and large
Sieves (colanders) in three sizes: small, medium, and large
Salad spinner or flour sack towels for drying salad
Vegetable peeler
Sharp knives:
   4-inch paring knife
   6-inch utility/sandwich knife
   8- or 9-inch chef's knife
   Steel rod or whetstone to sharpen the knives
   Cleaver

Cast-iron frying pan(s)
Long tongs
Wooden cutting board or chopping block
Ladle big enough to dish out all the soup you're going to be
  making
Can opener

Optional:
Measuring cups
Small bullet or mini-prep food processor
Food scale
Calorie-counter book
Whisk
Microplane grater
Lemon reamer or citrus squeezer

Appendix Four

Activity Ideas

No matter what you do, make sure it's fun. One step at a time, start down the road to a healthier life.

1. Walk every day with someone you love.

2. Take the whole family out for a quick walk after dinner.

3. Dance around the living room to music.

4. Put together a group of four friends. Get together once a week to exercise to an aerobics video, and then eat a healthy meal.

5. Take a belly dance class.

6. Have a friend teach you a new dance: hip-hop or the Lindy, depending on their age.

7. Organize a weekly dance party at your house or apartment.

8. Kick a soccer ball around with the kids.

9. Find an exercise bike on Craigslist and put it in the middle of your living room.

10. Call your cousin, the bodybuilder, and have him or her teach you how to lift weights at the gym.

11. Scour the Salvation Army for old aerobics tapes. Do one on the days you don't go for a walk.

12. Bike.

13. Swim.

14. Cross-country ski.

15. Make gym dates with a friend instead of dinner and a movie.

16. Play badminton. Portable sets are available for sale over the Internet. Bring the set to the next family picnic, so everyone can join in the activity instead of sitting around eating. It isn't as hard on the knees as tennis.

17. Instead of cruise vacations, take an active vacation that involves walking around new cities or national parks.

18. Babysit a friend's two-year-old son.

Appendix Five

The Diet

1. Walk or exercise every day, or at least five times a week. Exercise helps you lose belly fat.

2. Make new friends that are into health and fitness.

3. Eat three meals and one or two snacks every day.

4. Spread your food out throughout the day, using 100 calories per hour as a template. Don't starve during the day and binge at dinner.

5. Avoid all foods with high fructose corn syrup, including soda and sweetened soft drinks.

6. Avoid all food with trans fats.

7. By eliminating HFCS and trans fats, you'll essentially be eliminating processed foods.

8. Cut way down on the starches you eat.

9. Eat a dark green leafy vegetable every day.

10. Aim for ten servings of fruits and vegetables every day. If ten are too hard, five are fine.

11. Make sure you eat healthy fats every day. Don't eat a low-fat diet.

12. Don't spend money on weight-loss supplements.

13. Chocolate is allowed, but in moderation.

14. Organize your life and your kitchen.

15. Get some sunshine or take a vitamin D supplement.

16. Eat when you are hungry.

17. Sleep when you are tired.

18. Look back to your heritage for ideas on a healthy diet and lifestyle.

19. Always remember that you are beautiful. Don't let anyone make you feel otherwise. Tell them that fifty is the new thirty, and big is the new beautiful.

Appendix Six

Mercury Content of Seafood

M ercury is a naturally occurring chemical found in the environment. It's the silver-gray liquid in old-fashioned thermometers and blood pressure cuffs. Those old-fashioned thermometers and blood pressure cuffs are being phased out because mercury is so toxic. When these items break, they are discarded and end up in landfills, and ultimately in the oceans.

Thermometers in landfills are really not the root of mercury pollution in the oceans though. The real problem is the mercury released in the air from industrial pollution. When mercury falls into the oceans, it collects in bacteria and on seaweed and plankton. Small fish eat the plankton. Bigger fish eat the smaller fish and so on. At each point up the food chain, the mercury (actually, it's a form of mercury called methylmercury) accumulates in higher and higher concentrations. The largest fish with the longest life spans, and people, have the highest concentrations of mercury.

If you're pregnant, the nutrients found in seafood are important to the brain of the developing fetus, so you're between a rock and a hard place. On the one hand, you want to include seafood in your diet, but you need to choose carefully to avoid seafood high in mercury. Mercury can cause a whole array of developmental disabilities in a developing fetus.

For more information on the mercury content of fish, go to www.epa.gov/waterscience/fish. However, there is some concern that the EPA data is not current. I recommend the Environmental Working Group web site at www.ewg.org for information on mercury. The EWG is a watchdog organization, which monitors pollutants (in cosmetics, food, and the environment) affecting our health. I strongly recommend you visit this site just on general principle. Another site is www.gotmercury.org. This site has a calculator, so you can input the type of fish and the amount you're going to eat, and it will give you the mercury content. It even has a mercury calculator in Spanish. The Department of Health web site for your state offers another resource. The state web sites may have a list of the mercury content of locally caught fish in your area.

Don't just go by my list. The information keeps changing. The web sites will have very specific information as to how much you can eat of each particular fish, and how often.

Seafood Low in Mercury[1]	Seafood Moderate in Mercury	Seafood High in Mercury (Avoid When Pregnant):
Anchovies	Atlantic Croaker	Canned Albacore Tuna
Clams	Catfish	Grouper
Crawfish/Crayfish	Canned Light Tuna	Halibut
Herring	Cod	King Mackerel
Oysters	Crab	Largemouth Bass
Pollack	Flounder	Marlin
Sardines	Haddock	Pike
Shrimp	Mackerel	Sea Bass
Tilapia	Mussels	Shark
Whiting	Perch (Ocean or White)	Swordfish
Wild Salmon[2]	Scallops	Tilefish
	Shad	Tuna Steaks
	Sole	
	Squid/Calamari	
	Trout	
	Whitefish	

---

1. Fish sticks don't have much mercury, but they contain trans fats and pesticides.
2. Wild salmon is very expensive, when you can find it. Farmed salmon is low in mercury, but it contains high levels of PCBs (polychlorinated biphenyls), which are toxic to all living creatures. Farmed salmon has thirteen times more pollutants than wild salmon.

Appendix Seven

Green Powdered Fruit and Vegetable Extracts

Your best bet for finding these extracts might be the Internet, especially if you don't live in a large metropolitan area. Some of the vitamin supply web sites will have a whole variety on sale. You could pick and choose among the choices.

These powders are expensive. A jar can cost between twenty-five and forty-five dollars for thirty servings. If you calculate the cost, they end up setting you back anywhere between twenty-five and seventy-five cents per serving. They cost so much because it takes a lot of broccoli, kale, papaya, pineapple, spinach, barley, wheat grass, beets, apple, and alfalfa to dehydrate down to a scoop of this powder.

Whole Foods has a variety of these supplements in stock as well. When I first started going to Whole Foods after they opened their first store in New York City, they did not carry these extracts. Then, after a couple of years, they had a brand or two in stock. Now, they have so many that I have trouble choosing between them. Be forewarned, Whole Foods is not cheap. Some people jokingly call it, "Whole Paycheck." The last time I was in a GNC a few years ago, there was only one brand in stock. Now they too have a whole variety in stock. Through the years, more and more brands have become available as people discover these green powders.

Be sure to choose an organic brand, since pesticides and herbicides would get concentrated into the powder as well.

Some of the choices on the market include:

Gary Null's Green Stuff (www.garynull.com)
Barlean's Greens (www.barleans.com)
ProGreens from NutriCology (www.nutricology.com)
Greens Today from Nature's Answer (www.naturesanswer.com)
Macro Greens (www.macrolifenaturals.com)
Green Vibrance from Vibrant Health (www.vibranthealth.us)
Berry Green from New Chapter Inc. (www.newchapter.com)
Green Edge from Country Life (www.country-life.com)
Magma from Green Foods (www.greenfoods.com)
Perfect Food from Garden of Life (www.gardenoflife.com)
All One Green Phyto Base from Nutritech (www.all-one.com)
Greens Blend from Whole Foods
Beyond Greens from Udo's Choice (www.udoerasmus.com)

Udo Erasmus is a famous researcher who specializes in healthy fats.

Further Reading and Resources

The ‡ symbol indicates that a summary of the medical article, in layperson's terms, can be found on my web site.

Get Organized

Bittman, Mark. "A No-Frills Kitchen Still Cooks." *New York Times*, May 9, 2007.

———. "Fresh Start for a New Year? Let's Begin in the Kitchen." *New York Times*, January 7, 2009.

Lewine, Edward. "Craft House (An Interview with Tom Colicchio)." *New York Times Magazine*, May 3, 2009.

Get Motivated!

Al-Anon/Alateen. http://www.al-anon.org.

Beattie, Melody. *Co-Dependent No More: How to Stop Controlling Others and Start Caring for Yourself.* Center City, MN: Hazelden Press, 1992.

Brockway, Laurie Sue. *A Goddess Is a Girl's Best Friend.* New York: Perigee Press, 2002.

———. The Goddess Pages. http://www.goddessfriends.com.

Henig, Robin Marantz. "Losing the Weight Stigma: A Social Movement Argues That You Can Be Healthy No Matter How Fat You Are." *New York Times Magazine,* October 5, 2008.

Norwood, Robin. *Women Who Love Too Much: When You Keep Wishing and Hoping He'll Change.* New York: Pocket Books, 1985.

Overeaters Anonymous. http://www.oa.org.

Fats, Lipids, and Oils

CalorieLab. "GM Soybean Oil to Aid in Reducing Trans Fat." http://calorielab.com/news/2005/12/10/gm-soybean-oil-to-aid-in-reducing-trans-fat/.

Erasmus, Udo. *Fats That Heal, Fats That Kill: The Complete Guide to Fats, Oils, Cholesterol and Human Health.* Burnaby, BC: Alive Books, 1993.

Esmailzadeh, A., and A. Azadbakht. "Home Use of Vegetable Oils, Markers of Systemic Inflammation, and Endothelial Dysfunction Among Women." *American Journal of Clinical Nutrition* 88, no. 4 (2008): 913–921.

Jakobsen, M. U., E. J. O'Reilly, B. L. Heitmann, M. A. Pereira, K. Bälter, G. E. Fraser, U. Goldbourt, et al. "Major Types of Dietary Fat and Risk of Coronary Heart Disease: A Pooled Analysis of 11 Cohort Studies." *American Journal of Clinical Nutrition* 89, no. 5 (2009): 1425–1432.

Knopp, R. H., and B. M. Retzlaff. "Saturated Fat Prevents Coronary Heart Disease? An American Paradox." *American Journal of Clinical Nutrition* 80, no. 5 (2004): 1102–1103.

Mente, A., L. de Konig, H. S. Shannon, and S. S. Anand. "A Systemic Review of the Evidence Supporting a Causal Link between Dietary Factors and Coronary Heart Disease." *Archives of Internal Medicine* 169, no. 7 (2009): 659–669.

Mihm, Stephen. "Does Eating Salmon Lower the Murder Rate? What Omega-3 Fatty Acids Might Do for Violent Behavior." *New York Times Magazine,* April 16, 2006.

Mozaffarian, D., E. B. Rimm, and D. M. Herrington. "Dietary Fats, Carbohydrate, and Progression of Coronary Atherosclerosis in Postmenopausal Women." *American Journal of Clinical Nutrition* 80, no. 5 (2004): 1175–1184.

Schwartz, G. J. "Obesity, Dietary Fat and Satiety: Role of the Lipid Messenger OEA." Lecture, the Mount Sinai Medical Center Weight Management Grand Rounds, New York, NY, February 23, 2009.

Taubes, Gary. "What If It's All Been a Big Fat Lie?" *New York Times Magazine,* July 7, 2002.

Tierney, John. "Diet and Fat: A Severe Case of Mistaken Consensus." *New York Times,* October 9, 2007.

HFCS and Sugar

Dhingra, R., L. Sullivan, P. F. Jacques, T. J. Wang, C. S. Fox, J. B. Meigs, R. B. D'Agostino, J. Michael Gaziano, and R. S. Vasan. "Soft Drink Consumption and Risk of Developing Cardiometabolic Risk Factors and the Metabolic Syndrome in Middle-Aged Adults in the Community." *Circulation* 116, no. 5 (2007): 480–488.

Feinglos, M. N., and S. E. Totten. "Are You What You Eat or How Much You Eat? The Case of Type 2 Diabetes." *Archives of Internal Medicine* 168, no. 14 (2008): 1485–1486.

Fung, T. T., V. Malik, K. M. Rexrode, J. E. Mason, W. C. Willett, and F. B. Hu. "Sweetened Beverage Consumption and Risk of Coronary Heart Disease in Women." *American Journal of Clinical Nutrition* 89, no. 4 (2009): 1037–1042.

‡Lutsey, P. L., L. M. Steffen, and J. Stevens. "Dietary Intake and the Development of the Metabolic Syndrome: The Atherosclerosis Risk in Communities Study." *Circulation* 117, no. 6 (2008): 754–761.

Nettleton, J. A., P. L. Lutsey, Y. Wang, J. A. Lima, D. Michos, and D. R. Jacobs Jr. "Diet Soda Intake and Risk of Incident Metabolic Syndrome and Type 2 Diabetes in the Multi-Ethnic Study of Atherosclerosis (MESA)." *Diabetes Care* 32, no. 4 (2009): 688–694.

‡Palmer, J. E., D. A. Boggs, S. Krishman, F. S. Hu, M. Singer, and L. Rosenberg. "Sugar-Sweetened Beverages and the Incidence of Type 2 Diabetes in African American Women." *Archives of Internal Medicine* 168, no. 14 (2008): 1487–1492.

Advanced Glycation End-Products

Moreau, R. "Browning: The Dark Side of Sugar." Linus Pauling Institute. http://lpi.oregonstate.edu/fw04/browning.html.

Peppa, M., J. Uribarri, and H. Vlassara. "Glucose, Advanced Glycation End Products, and Diabetes Complications: What Is New and What Works." *Clinical Diabetes* 21, no. 4 (2003): 186–187.

Ramasamy, R., S. J. Vannucci, S. S. D. Yan, K. Herold, S. F. Yan, and A. M. Schmidt. "Advanced Glycation End Products and RAGE: A Common Thread in Aging, Diabetes, Neurodegeneration, and Inflammation." *Glycobiology* 15, no. 7 (March 10, 2005). http://glycob.oxfordjournals.org/cgi/content/full/15/7/16R.

Vlassara, H. "Dietary Glycoxidants: A Driving Force in the Metabolic Syndrome and Diabetes: Can a Diet Low in Advanced Glycation End-Products Be the Answer?" Lecture, the Mount Sinai Medical Center Weight Management Grand Rounds, New York, NY, December 10, 2007.

Vlassara, H., and J. Uribarri. "Glycoxidative Stress and the Metabolic Syndrome: Can a Diet Low in Advanced Glycation End-Products Be the Answer?" Lecture, the Mount Sinai Medical Center Weight Management Grand Rounds, New York, NY, February 27, 2006.

Glycemic Index Lists

Glassman, Greg. "Glycemic Index." *The CrossFit Journal* no. 3 (November 2002). http://www.crossfit.com/journal/library/GlycemicNov02.pdf.

Mendosa, David. "Revised International Table of Glycemic Index (GI) and Glycemic Load (GL) Values—2008." Mendosa.com. http://www.mendosa.com/gilists.htm.

Diets and Healthy Eating

Agatston, Arthur. *The South Beach Diet.* New York: Rodale Books, 2003.

Anderson, C. A. M., and L. J. Appel. "Dietary Modification and CVD Prevention: A Matter of Fat." *Journal of the American Medical Association* 295, no. 6 (2006): 693–694.

Atkins, Robert C. *Dr. Atkins' New Diet Revolution.* Revised edition. New York: M. Evans and Company, 2003.

Beresford, S. A. A., K. C. Johnson, C. Ritenbaugh, N. L. Lasser, L. G. Snetselaar, H. R. Black, G. L. Anderson, et al. "Low-Fat Dietary Pattern and Risk of Colorectal Cancer: The Women's Health Initiative Randomized Controlled Dietary Modification Trial." *Journal of the American Medical Association* 295, no. 6 (2006): 643–654.

Buzdar, A. U. "Dietary Modification and Risk of Breast Cancer." *Journal of the American Medical Association* 295, no. 6 (2006): 691–692.

Clower, Will. *The Fat Fallacy: The French Diet Secrets to Permanent Weight Loss.* New York: Three River Press, 2003.

Ebbeling, C. B., M. M. Leidig, H. A. Feldman, M. M. Lovesky, and D. S. Ludwig. "Effects of a Low-Glycemic Load vs. Low-Fat Diet in Obese Young Adults: A Randomized Trial." *Journal of the American Medical Association* 297, no. 19 (2007): 2092–2102.

Fallon, Sally, and Mary G. Enig. "Myths and Truths About Soy." The Weston A. Price Foundation. http://westonaprice.org/mythstruths/mtsoy.html.

———. "Soy: The Dark Side of America's Favorite 'Health Food.'" The Weston A. Price Foundation. http://www.westonaprice.org/soy/darkside.html.

Gardner, C. D., A. Kiazand, S. Alhassan, S. Kim, R. S. Stafford, R. R. Balise, H. C. Kraemer, and A. C. King. "Comparison of the Atkins, Zone, Ornish and LEARN Diets for Change in Weight and Related Risk Factors among Overweight Premenopausal Women. The A to Z Weight Loss Study: A Randomized Trial." *Journal of the American Medical Association* 297, no. 9 (2007): 969–977.

Guiliano, Mireille. *French Women Don't Get Fat.* New York: Knopf, 2004.

Howard, B. V., J. E. Manson, M. L. Stefanick, S. A. Beresford, G. Frank, B. Jones, R. J. Rodabough, et al. "Low-Fat Dietary Pattern and Weight Change Over 7 Years: The Women's Health Initiative Dietary Modification Trial." *Journal of the American Medical Association* 295, no. 1 (2006): 39–49.

Howard, B. V., L. Van Horn, J. Hsia, J. A. E. Manson, M. L. Stefanick, S. Wassertheil-Smoller, L. H. Kuller, et al. "Low-Fat Dietary Pattern and Risk of Cardiovascular Disease: The Women's Health Initiative Randomized Controlled Dietary Modification Trial." *Journal of the American Medical Association* 295, no. 6 (2006): 655–666.

McMillan-Price, J., P. Petocz, F. Atkinson, K. O'Neill, S. Samman, K. Steinbeck, I. Caterson, and J. Brand-Miller. "Comparison of 4 Diets of Varying Glycemic Load on Weight Loss and Cardiovascular Risk Reduction in Overweight and Obese Young Adults: A Randomized Controlled Trial." *Archives of Internal Medicine* 166, no. 14 (2006): 1446–1475.

Nestle, Marion, and L. Beth Dixon. *Taking Sides: Clashing Views on Controversial Issues in Food and Nutrition.* Guilford, CT: McGraw-Hill, 2004.

Ornish, Dean. *Dean Ornish's Program for Reversing Heart Disease.* New York: Ballantine Books, 1990.

‡Phillips, S. A., J. W. Jurva, A. Q. Syed, J. P. Kulinski, J. Pleuss, R. G. Hoffman, and D. D. Gutterman. "Benefit of Low-Fat Over Low-Carbohydrate Diet on Endothelial Health in Obesity." *Hypertension* 51, no. 2 (2008): 376–380.

Planck, Nina. *Real Food: What to Eat and Why.* New York: Bloomsbury, 2006.

Pollan, Michael. *In Defense of Food: An Eater's Manifesto.* New York: The Penguin Press, 2008.

Prentice, R. L., B. Caan, R. T. Chlebowski, R. Patterson, L. H. Kuller, J. K. Ockene, K. L. Margolis, et al. "Low-Fat Dietary Pattern and Risk of Invasive Breast Cancer: The Women's Health Initiative Randomized Controlled Dietary Modification Trial." *Journal of the American Medical Association* 295, no. 6 (2006): 629–642.

Sears, Barry. *The Anti-Aging Zone.* New York: Regan Books, 1999.

———. *Enter the Zone.* New York: Collins Living, 1995.

‡Shai, I., D. Schwarzfuchs, Y. Henkin, D. R. Shahar, S. Witkow, I. Greenberg, R. Golan, et al. "Weight Loss with a Low-Carbohydrate, Mediterranean, or Low-Fat Diet." *New England Journal of Medicine* 359, no. 3 (2008): 229–241.

Steinberg, Francene M. "Soybeans or Soymilk: Does It Make a Difference for Cardiovascular Protection? Does It Even Matter?" *American Journal of Clinical Nutrition* 85, no. 4 (2007): 927–928.

Taubes, Gary. *Good Calories, Bad Calories.* New York: Knopf, 2007.

‡Tinker, Lesley F., Denise E. Bonds, Karen L. Margolis, J. E. Manson, B. V. Howard, J. Larsen, M. G. Perri, et al. "Low-Fat Dietary Pattern and Risk of Treated Diabetes Mellitus in Postmenopausal Women: The Women's Health Initiative Dietary Modification Trial." *Archives of Internal Medicine* 168, no. 14 (2008): 1500–1511.

Mediterranean Diet
Bautista, M. C., and M. M. Engler. "The Mediterranean Diet: Is It Cardioprotective?" *Progress in Cardiovascular Nursing* 20, no. 2 (2005): 70–76.

Blackburn, Henry. "On the Trail of Heart Attacks in Seven Countries." University of Minnesota. http://www.epi.umn.edu/research/7countries/index.shtm.

Gaifyllia, Nancy. "Wild and Cultivated Greens in Greek Recipes." About.com. http://greekfood.about.com/od/discovergreekfood/a/wild_greens.htm.

Jiang, R., D. R. Jacobs, E. Mayer-Davis, M. Szklo, D. Herrington, N. S. Jenny, R. Kronmal, and R. G. Barr. "Nut and Seed Consumption and Inflammatory Markers in the Multi-Ethnic Study of Atherosclerosis." *American Journal of Epidemiology* 163, no. 3 (2006): 222–231.

Kalliopi, K., C. Papamichael, E. Karatzis, T. G. Papaioannou, P. Th. Voidonikola, G. D. Vamvakou, J. Lekakis, and A. Zampelas. "Postprandial Improvement of Endothelial Function by Red Wine and Olive Oil Antioxidants: A Synergistic Effect of

Components of the Mediterranean Diet." *Journal of the American College of Nutrition* 27, no. 4 (2008): 448–453.

Knoops, K. T. B., L. C. P. G. M. de Groot, D. Kromhout, A.-E. Perrin, O. Moreiras-Varela, A. Menotti, and W. A. van Staveren. "Mediterranean Diet, Lifestyle Factors, and 10-year Mortality in Elderly European Men and Women: The HALE Project." *Journal of the American Medical Association* 292, no. 12 (2004): 1433–1439.

Martinez-González, M. A., C. de la Fuente-Arrillaga, J. M. Nunez-Cordoba, F. J. Basterra-Gortari, J. J. Beunza, Z. Vazquez, S. Benito, A. Tortosa, and M. Rastrollo. "Adherence to Mediterranean Diet and Risk of Developing Diabetes: Prospective Cohort Study." *BMJ* 336, no. 7657 (2008): 1348–1351.

Mitrou, P. N., V. Kipnis, A. C. M. Thiébaut, J. Reedy, A. F. Subar, E. Wirfält, A. Flood, et al. "Mediterranean Dietary Pattern and Prediction of All-Cause Mortality in a US Population: Results from the NIH-AARP Diet and Health Study." *Archives of Internal Medicine* 167, no. 22 (2007): 2461–2468.

Salas-Salvadó, J., J. Fernández-Ballart, E. Ros, M.-A. Martinez-Gonzalez, M. Fitó, R. Estruch, D. Corella, et al. "Effect of a Mediterranean Diet Supplemented with Nuts on Metabolic Syndrome Status: One-Year Results of PREDIMED Randomized Trial." *Archives of Internal Medicine* 68, no. 22 (2008): 2449–2458.

Simopoulos, A. P. "Evolutionary Aspects of Diet, Essential Fatty Acids and Cardiovascular Disease." *European Heart Journal Supplements* 3 (2001): D8–21.

———. "The Mediterranean Diets: What is So Special about the Diet of Greece? The Scientific Evidence." *Journal of Nutrition* 131, no. 11 (2001): S3065–S3073.

———. "Omega-3 Fatty Acids and Antioxidants in Edible Wild Plants." *Biological Research* 37, no. 2 (2004): 263–277.

Sofi, F., F. Cesari, R. Abbate, G. F. Gensini, and A. Casini. "Adherence to Mediterranean Diet and Health Status: Meta-Analysis." *BMJ* 337 (2008). http://www.bmj.com/cgi/content/full/337/sep11_2/a1344.

Antioxidants, Multivitamins, and Supplements
Agricultural Research Service. "Nutrient Data Laboratory." http://www.ars.usda.gov/nutrientdata.

Antioxidants
Barger, J. L., T. Kayo, J. M. Vann, E. B. Arias, J. Wang, T. A. Hacker, Y. Wang, et al. "A Low Dose of Dietary Resveratrol Partially Mimics Calorie Restriction and Retards Aging Parameters in Mice." *PLoS ONE* 3, no. 6 (2008). http://www.plosone.org/article/info%3Adoi%2F10.1371%2Fjournal.pone.0002264.

Bjelakovic, G., and C. Gluud. "Surviving Antioxidant Supplements." *Journal of the National Cancer Institute* 99, no. 10 (2007): 742–3.

Bliss, Rosalie Marion. "Beneficial Compounds in Cinnamon Spice Up Insulin Sensitivity." Agricultural Research Service. http://www.ars.usda.gov/IS/pr/2004/040419.htm.

Heinonen, O. P., and D. Albanes. "The Effect of Vitamin E and Beta-Carotene on the Incidence of Lung Cancer and Other Cancers in Male Smokers." *New England Journal of Medicine* 330, no.15 (1994): 1029–1035.

Joseph, J. A., B. Shukitt-Hale, N. A. Denisova, D. Bielinksi, A. Martin, J. J. McEwen, and P. C. Bickford. "Reversals of Age-Related Declines in Neuronal Signal Transduction, Cognitive, and Motor Behavioral Deficits with Blueberry, Spinach, or Strawberry Dietary Supplementation." *Journal of Neuroscience* 19, no. 18 (1999): 8114–8121.

Malaguarnera, M., M. Vacante, T. Avitabile, M. Malaguarnera, L. Cammalleri, and M. Motta. "L-Carnitine Supplementation Reduces Oxidized LDL Cholesterol in Patients with Diabetes." *American Journal of Clinical Nutrition* 89, no.1 (2009): 71–76.

Nutrient Data Laboratory, Beltsville Human Nutrition Resource Center, Agricultural Research Service, U.S. Department of Agriculture. *USDA Database for the Proanthocyanidin Content of Selected Foods.* Beltsville, MD: Nutrient Data Laboratory, 2004. http://www.nal.usda.gov/fnic/foodcomp/Data/PA/PA.pdf.

Nutrient Data Laboratory, Food Composition Laboratory, Beltsville Human Nutrition Resource Center, Agricultural Research Service, U.S. Department of Agriculture. *USDA Database for the Flavonoid Content of Selected Foods, Release 2.1.* Beltsville, MD: Nutrient Data Laboratory, 2007. http://www.nal.usda.gov/fnic/foodcomp/Data/Flav/Flav02-1.pdf.

Seymore, E. M., A. A. M. Singer, M. R. Bennik, R. V. Parikh, A. Kirakosyan, P. B. Kaufman, and S. F. Bolling. "Chronic Intake of a Phytochemical-Enriched Diet Reduces Cardiac Fibrosis and Diastolic Dysfunction Caused by Prolonged Salt-Sensitive Hypertension." *Journal of Gerontology Series A* 63 (2008): 1034–1042.

Calcium

Bolland, M. J., A. Barber, R. N. Doughty, B. Mason, A. Horne, R. Ames, G. D. Gamble, A. Grey, and I. R. Reid. "Vascular Events in Healthy Older Women Receiving Calcium Supplementation: Randomized Controlled Trial." *BMJ* 336, no. 7638 (2008): 262–266.

Daniel, Kaayla T. "Why Broth is Beautiful—'Essential' Roles for Proline, Glycine and Gelatin." Weston A. Price Foundation. http://www.westonaprice.org/foodfeatures/brothisbeautiful.html.

Fallon, Sally. "Broth is Beautiful." Weston A. Price Foundation. http://westonaprice.org/foodfeatures/broth.html.

Napoli, N., J. Thompson, R. Civitelli, and R. C. Armamento-Villareal. "Effects of Dietary Calcium Compared with Calcium Supplements on Estrogen Metabolism and Bone Mineral Density." *American Journal of Clinical Nutrition* 85, no. 5 (2007): 1428–1433.

Park, Y., M. F. Leitzmann, A. F. Subar, A. Hollenbeck, and A. Schatzkin. "Dairy Food, Calcium, and Risk of Cancer in the NIH-AARP Diet and Health Study." *Archives of Internal Medicine* 169, no. 4 (2009): 391–401.

U.S. Department of Agriculture. "USDA National Nutrient Database for Standard Reference, Release 17: Calcium, Ca (mg) Content of Selected Foods per Common Measure, sorted alphabetically." http://www.nal.usda.gov/fnic/foodcomp/Data/SR17/wtrank/sr17a301.pdf.

Varemma, M., L. Binelli, S. Casari, F. Zucchi, and L. Sinigaglia. "Effects of Dietary Calcium Intake on Body Weight and Prevalence of Osteoporosis in Early Postmenopausal Women." *American Journal of Clinical Nutrition* 86, no. 3 (2007): 639–644.

Chocolate

‡Balzar, J., T. Rassaf, C. Heiss, P. Kleinbongard, T. Lauer, M. Merx, N. Heussen, et al. "Sustained Benefits in Vascular Function Through Flavanol-Containing Cocoa in Medicated Diabetic Patients." *Journal of the American College of Cardiology* 51, no. 22 (2008): 2141–2149.

‡Buijsse, B., E. J. M. Feskens, F. J. Kok, and D. Kromhout. "Cocoa Intake, Blood Pressure, and Cardiovascular Mortality: The Zutphen Elderly Study." *Archives of Internal Medicine* 166, no. 4 (2006): 411–417.

Gertner, Jon. "Eat Chocolate, Live Longer?" *The New York Times Magazine,* October 10, 2004.

‡Taubert, D., R. Roesen, C. Lehmann, N. Jung, and E. Schömig. "Effects of Low Habitual Cocoa Intake on Blood Pressure and Bioactive Nitric Oxide: A Randomized Controlled Trial." *Journal of the American Medical Association* 298, no. 1 (2007): 49–60.

Taubert, D., R. Roesen, and E. Schömig. "Effect of Cocoa and Tea Intake on Blood Pressure: A Meta-Analysis." *Archives of Internal Medicine* 167, no. 7 (2007): 626–634.

Multivitamins and Supplements
Bjelakovic, G., D. Nikolova, L. L. Gluud, R. G. Simonetti, and C. Gluud. "Mortality in Randomized Trials of Antioxidant Supplements for Primary and Secondary Prevention: Systematic Review and Meta-Analysis." *Journal of the American Medical Association* 297, no. 8 (2007): 842–857.

Cole, B. F., J. A. Baron, R. S. Sandler, R. W. Haile, D. J. Ahnen, R. S. Bresalier, G. McKeown-Eyssen, et al. "Folic Acid for the Prevention of Colorectal Adenomas." *Journal of the American Medical Association* 297, no. 21 (2007): 2351–2359.

Lawson K. A., M. E. Wright, A. Subar, T. Mouw, A. Hollenbeck, A. Achatzkin, and M. F. Leitzmann. "Multivitamin Use and Risk of Prostate Cancer in the National Institutes of Health-AARP Diet and Health Study." *Journal of the National Cancer Institute* 99, no. 10 (2007): 754–764.

Omenn G. S., G. E. Goodman, M. D. Thornquist, J. Balmes, M. R. Cullen, and A. Glass. "Risk Factors for Lung Cancer and for Intervention Effects in CARET, the Beta-Carotene and Retinol Efficacy Trial." *Journal of the National Cancer Institute* 88, no. 21 (1996): 1550–1559.

Parker-Pope, T. "Vitamin Pills: A False Hope?" *New York Times,* February 17, 2009.

Sesso, H. D., J. E. Buring, W. G. Christen, T. Kurth, C. Belanger, J. MacFadyen, V. Bubes, J. E. Manson, R. J. Glynn, and J. M. Gaziano. "Vitamins E and C in the Prevention of Cardiovascular Disease in Men: The Physicians' Health Study II Randomized Controlled Trial." *Journal of the American Medical Association* 300, no. 18 (2008): 2123–2133.

Ulrich, C. M., and J. D. Potter. "Folate and Cancer—Timing is Everything." *Journal of the American Medical Association* 297, no. 21 (2007): 2408–2409.

USDA/ARS Children's Nutrition Research Center at Baylor College of Medicine. "Fortify Your Folate Levels Before Becoming Pregnant." http://www.bcm.edu/cnrc/consumer/archives/fortify-folate.htm.

Zhang, S. M., N. R. Cook, C. M. Albert, J. M. Gaziano, J. E. Buring, and J. E. Manson. "Effect of Combined Folic Acid, Vitamin B_6, and Vitamin B_{12} on Cancer Risk in Women: A Randomized Trial." *Journal of the American Medical Association* 300, no. 17 (2008): 2012–2021.

Vitamin D and Bone Health

Autier, P., and S. Gandini. "Vitamin D Supplementation and Total Mortality. A Meta-Analysis of Randomized Controlled Trials." *Archives of Internal Medicine* 176, no. 16 (2007): 1730–1737.

Brody, Jane E. "An Oldie Vies for Nutrient of the Decade." *New York Times,* February 19, 2008.

Caan, B., M. Neuhouser, A. Aragaki, C. B. Lewis, R. Jackson, M. S. LeBoff, K. L. Margolis, et al. "Calcium Plus Vitamin D Supplementation and the Risk of Postmenopausal Weight Gain." *Archives of Internal Medicine* 167, no. 9 (2008): 893–902.

‡Cockayne, A., J. Adamson, S. Lanham-New, M. J. Schrer, S. Gilbody, and D. J. Torgerson. "Vitamin K and the Prevention of Fractures: Systematic Review and Meta-Analysis of

Randomized Controlled Trials." *Archives of Internal Medicine* 166, no. 12 (2006): 1256–1261.

Dobnig, H., S. Pilz, H. Scharnagl, W. Renner, U. Seelhorst, B. Wellnitz, J. Kinkeldei, B. O. Boehm, G. Weihrauch, and W. Maerz. "Independent Association of Low Serum 25-Hydroxyvitamin D and 1.25-Dihydroxyvitamin D Levels with All-Cause and Cardiovascular Mortality." *Archives of Internal Medicine* 168, no. 12 (2008): 1340–1349.

Fallon, Sally, and Mary G. Enig. "Vitamin A, Vitamin D & Cod-liver Oil: Some Clarifications." The Weston A. Price Foundation. http://www.westonaprice.org/basicnutrition/cod-liver-oil-menu.html.

Forman, J. P., E. Giovannucci, M. D. Holmes, H. A. Bischoff-Ferrari, S. S. Tworoger, W. C. Willett, and G. C. Curhan. "Plasma 25-Hydroxyvitamin D Levels and Risk of Incident Hypertension." *Hypertension* 49, no. 5 (2007):1063–1069.

Forouhi, N. G., J. Luan, A. Cooper, B. J. Boucher, and N. J. Wareman. "Baseline Serum 25-Hydroxy Vitamin D is Predictive of Future Glycemic Status and Insulin Resistance." *Diabetes* 57, no. 10 (2008): 2619–2625.

Ginde, A. A., J. M. Mansbach, and C. A. Camargo. "Association Between Serum 25-Hydroxyvitamin D Level and Upper Respiratory Tract Infection in the Third National Health and Nutrition Survey." *Archives of Internal Medicine* 169, no. 4 (2009): 384–390.

Giovannucci, E. "Can Vitamin D Reduce Total Mortality?" *Archives of Internal Medicine* 176, no. 16 (2007): 1709–1710.

Giovannucci, G. "Expanding Roles of Vitamin D." *Journal of Clinical Endocrinology and Metabolism* 94, no. 2 (2009): 418–420.

Giovannucci, G., Y. Liu, B. W. Hollis, and E. B. Rimm. "25-Hydroxyvitamin D and Risk of Myocardial Infarction in Men." *Archives of Internal Medicine* 168, no. 11 (2008): 1174–1180.

Hathcock, J. N., A. Shao, R. Vieth, and R. Heaney. "Risk Assessment for Vitamin D3." *American Journal of Clinical Nutrition* 85, no. 1 (2007): 6–18.

Hsia, J., G. Heiss, H. Ren, M. Allison, N. C. Dolan, P. Greenland, S. R. Heckbert, et al. "Calcium/Vitamin D Supplementation and Cardiovascular Events." *Circulation* 115, no. 7 (2007): 846–854.

Martins, D., M. Wolf, D. Pan, A. Zadshir, N. Tareen, R. Thadhani, A. Felsenfeld, B. Levine, R. Mehrotra, and K. Norris. "Prevalence of Cardiovascular Risk Factors and the Serum Levels of 25-Hydroxyvitamin D in the United States: Data From the Third National Health and Nutrition Examination Survey." *Archives of Internal Medicine* 167, no. 11 (2007): 1159–1165.

‡Melamed, M. M., E. D. Michos, W. Post, and B. Astor. "25-Hydroxyvitamin D Levels and the Risk of Mortality in the General Population." *Archives of Internal Medicine* 168, no. 15 (2008): 1629–1637.

Michos, E. D., and R. S. Blumenthal. "Vitamin D Supplementation and Cardiovascular Risk, Editorial." *Circulation* 115, no. 7 (2007): 827–828.

Mosekilde, L. "Vitamin D and the Elderly." *Clinical Endocrinology* 62, no. 3 (2005): 265–281.

Park, S.-Y., S. P. Murphy, L. R. Wilkens, A. M. Y. Nomura, B. E. Henderson, and L. N. Kolonel. "Calcium and Vitamin D Intake and Risk of Colorectal Cancer: The Multiethnic Cohort Study." *American Journal of Epidemiology* 165, no. 7 (2007): 784–793.

Pittas, A. G., S. S. Harris, P. C. Stark, and B. Dawson-Hughes. "The Effects of Calcium and Vitamin D Supplementation on Blood Glucose and Markers of Inflammation in Nondiabetic Adults." *Diabetes Care* 30, no. 4 (2007): 980–986.

Pittas, A. G., J. Lau, F. B. Hu, and B. Dawson-Hughs. "The Role of Vitamin D and Calcium in Type 2 Diabetes: A Systematic Review and Meta-Analysis." *Journal of Clinical Endocrinology & Metabolism* 92, no. 6 (2007): 2017–2029.

Vieth, R., H. Bischoff-Ferrari, B. J. Boucher, B. Dawson-Hughs, C. F. Garland, R. P. Heaney, M. F. Hollick, et al. "The Urgent Need to Recommend an Intake of Vitamin D That Is Effective." *American Journal of Clinical Nutrition* 85, no. 3 (2007): 649–650.

Metabolism

Henig, Robin Marantz. "Fat Factors." *New York Times Magazine,* August 8, 2006.

Kolata, Gina. *Rethinking Thin: The New Science of Weight Loss—and the Myths and Realities of Dieting.* New York: Picador, 2008.

———. "Genes Take Charge, and Diets Fall by the Wayside. *New York Times,* May 8, 2007.

Pool, Robert. *Fat: Fighting the Obesity Epidemic.* New York: Oxford University Press, 2001.

Sims, E. A. "Experimental Obesity, Dietary-Induced Thermogenesis, and Their Clinical Implications." *Clinics in Endocrinology and Metabolism* 5, no. 2 (1976): 377–395.

Brain and Hormone Effects on Metabolism, and Vice Versa

Alonso-Alonso, M. and A. Pascual-Leone. "The Right Brain Hypothesis for Obesity." *Journal of the American Medical Association* 297, no. 16 (2007): 1819–1822.

Convit, A. "Obesity in Children and Adults: Impact of Insulin Resistance on Brain Integrity." Lecture, annual NYU obesity prevention and management symposium, New York, NY, October 18, 2008.

Cummings, D. E., and K. E. Foster. "Ghrelin-Leptin Tango in Body-Weight Regulation." *Gastroenterology* 5 no. 124 (2003): 1532–1535.

Cummings, D. E., D. S. Weigle, R. S. Frayo, P. A. Breen, M. K. Ma, E. P. Dellinger, and J. Q. Purnell. "Plasma Ghrelin Levels After Diet-Induced Weight Loss or Gastric Bypass Surgery." *New England Journal of Medicine* 346, no. 21 (2002): 1623–30.

Egan, J. M., and R. F. Margolskee. "Taste Cells of the Gut and Gastrointestinal Chemosensation." *Molecular Interventions* 8, no. 2 (2008): 78–81.

Gold, S. M., I. Dziobek, V. Sweat, A. Tirsi, K. Rogers, H. Bruehl, W. Tsui, S. Richardson, E. Javier, and A. Convit. "Hippocampal Damage and Memory Impairments as Possible Early Brain Complications of Type 2 Diabetes." *Diabetologia* 50, no. 4 (2007): 711–719.

Keith, S. W., D. T. Redden, P. T. Katzmarzyk, M. M. Boggiano, E. C. Hanlon, R. M. Benca, D. Ruden, et al. "Putative Contributors to the Secular Increase in Obesity: Exploring the Roads Less Traveled." *International Journal of Obesity* 30, no. 11 (2006): 1585–1594.

Kohatsu, N. D., R. Tsai, T. Young, R. VanGilder, L. F. Burmeister, A. M. Stromquist, and J. A. Merchant. "Sleep Duration and Body Mass Index in a Rural Population." *Archives of Internal Medicine* 166, no. 16 (2006): 1701–1705.

Konturek, P. C., J. W. Konturek, M. Czesnikiewicz-Guzik, T. Brzozowski, E. Sito, and S. J. Konturek. "Neuro-Hormonal Control of Food Intake; Basic Mechanisms and Clinical

Implications." *Journal of Physiology and Pharmacology* 56, no. 6 (2005): S5–S25.

Taheri, S., L. Lin, D. Austin, T. Young, and E. Mignot. "Short Sleep Duration Is Associated with Reduced Leptin, Elevated Ghrelin, and Increased Body Mass Index." *PLoS Medicine* 1, no. 3 (2004): 62. http://dx.doi.org/10.1371%2Fjournal. pmed.0010062.

Exercise, Fitness, Obesity, and Longevity

Bravata, D. M., C. Smith-Spangler, V. Sundaram, A. L. Gienger, N. Lin, R. Lewis, C. D. Stave, I. Olkin, and J. R. Sirand. "Using Pedometers to Increase Physical Activity and Improve Health." *Journal of the American Medical Association* 298, no. 19 (2007): 2296–2304.

Buettner, Dan. *The Blue Zones: Lessons for Living Longer From the People Who Have Lived the Longest.* Washington, D.C.: National Geographic, 2008.

‡Chakravarty, E. F., H. B. Hubert, V. B. L., and J. F. Fries. "Reduced Disability and Mortality among Aging Runners: A 21-Year Longitudinal Study." *Archives of Internal Medicine* 168, no. 15 (2008): 1638–1646.

Cherkas, L. A., J. L. Hunkin, B. S. Kato, B. Richards, J. P. Gardner, G. L. Surdulescu, M. Kimuru, X. Lu, T. D. Spector, and A. Aviv. "The Association Between Physical Activity In Leisure Time and Leukocyte Telomere Length." *Archives of Internal Medicine* 168, no. 2 (2008): 154–158.

Church, T. S., C. P. Earnest, J. S. Skinner, and S. N. Blair. "Effects of Different Doses of Physical Activity on Cardiorespiratory Fitness among Sedentary, Overweight or Obese Postmenopausal Women with Elevated Blood Pressure." *Journal of the American Medical Association* 297, no. 19 (2007): 2081–2091.

Corcoran, M. P., S. Lamon-Fava, and R. A. Fielding. "Skeletal Muscle Lipid Deposition and Insulin Resistance: Effect of Dietary Fatty Acids and Exercise." *American Journal of Clinical Nutrition* 85, no. 3 (2007): 662–677.

Flegal, K. M., B. I. Graubard, D. F. Williamson, and M. H. Gail. "Cause-Specific Excess Deaths Associated With Underweight, Overweight, and Obesity." *Journal of the American Medical Association* 298, no. 17 (2007): 2028–2037.

Gregg, E. W., and J. M. Guralnik. "Is Disability Obesity's Price of Longevity?" *Journal of the American Medical Association* 298, no. 17 (2007): 2066–2067.

Hu, F. B. "Obesity and Mortality: Watch Your Waist, Not Just Your Weight." *Archives of Internal Medicine* 167, no. 9 (2007): 875–876.

‡Jakicic, J. M., B. H. Marcus, W. Lang, and C. Janney. "Effect of Exercise on 24-Month Weight Loss Maintenance in Over-weight Women." *Archives of Internal Medicine* 168, no. 14 (2008): 1550–1559.

Jeffrey, Allison N. "The Seeds Are Sown In Childhood: Insulin Resistance and the Global Epidemic of Type 2 Diabetes." In *Focus on Diabetes Mellitus Research*, edited by Ashley M. Ford, 144–168. Hauppauge, NY: Nova Biomedical Books, 2006.

Karelis, A. D., D. H. St-Pierre, F. Conus, R. Rabasa-Lhoret, and E. T. Poehlman. "Metabolic and Body Composition Factors in Subgroups of Obesity: What Do We Know." *Clinical Endocrinology and Metabolism* 89, no. 6 (2004): 2569–2575.

Kolata, Gina. "Chubby Gets a Second Look." *New York Times,* November 11, 2007.

———. "Causes of Death Are Linked to a Person's Weight." *New York Times,* November 7, 2007.

Landsberg, L. "Body Fat Distribution and Cardiovascular Risk: A Tale of 2 Sites." *Archives of Internal Medicine* 168, no. 15 (2008): 1607–1608.

Lee, I.-M. "Dose-Response Relation Between Physical Activity and Fitness: Even a Little is Good; More is Better." *Journal of the American Medical Association* 297, no. 19 (2007): 2137–2139.

Leitzmann, M. F., Y. Park, A. Blair, R. Ballard-Barbash, T. Mouw, A. R. Hollenbeck, and A. Schatzkin. "Physical Activity Recommendations and Decreased Risk of Mortality." *Archives of Internal Medicine* 167, no. 22 (2007): 2453–2460.

Satoru, K., K. Saito, S. Tanaka, M. Maki, Y. Yachi, M. Asumi, A. Sugowara, et al. "Cardiorespiratory Fitness as a Quantitative Predictor of All-Cause Mortality and Cardiovascular Events in Healthy Men and Women: A Meta-Analysis." *Journal of the American Medical Association* 301, no. 19 (2009): 2024–2035.

Stefan, N., K. Kantartzis, J. Machann, F. Schick, C. Thamer, K. Rittig, B. Balletshofer, F. Machicao, A. Fritsche, and H.-R. Häring. "Identification and Characterization of Metabolically Benign Obesity in Humans." *Archives of Internal Medicine* 168, no. 15 (2008): 1609–1616.

Sui, X., M. J. Lamonte, J. N. Laditka, J. W. Hardin, N. Chase, S. P. Hooker, and S. N. Blair. "Cardiorespiratory Fitness and Adiposity as Mortality Predictors in Older Adults." *Journal of the American Medical Association* 298, no. 21 (2007): 2507–2516.

Tolman, K. G., V. Fonseca, A. Dalpiaz, and M. H. Tan. "Spectrum of Liver Disease in Type 2 Diabetes and Management of Patients with Diabetes and Liver Disease." *Diabetes Care* 30, no. 3 (2007): 734–743.

Wang, X., T. You, L. Lenchik, and B. Nicklas. "Resting Energy Expenditure Changes with Weight Loss: Racial Differences."

Obesity (2009). http://www.nature.com/oby/journal/vaop/ncurrent/abs/oby2009163a.html.

‡Wildman, R. P., P. Muntner, K. Reynolds, A. P. McGinn, S. Rajpathak, J. Wylie-Rosett, and M. F. R. Sowers. "The Obese without Cardiometabolic Risk Factor Clustering and the Normal Weight with Cardiometabolic Risk Factor Clustering: Prevalence and Correlates of 2 Phenotypes among the US Population (NHANES 1999–2004)." *Archives of Internal Medicine* 168, no. 15 (2008): 1617–1624.

Organics and Plastics

Burke, Cindy. *To Buy or Not To Buy Organic.* New York: Marlowe and Company, 2007.

Burros, Marian. "The Customer Wants a Juicy Steak? Just Add Water." *New York Times*, August 9, 2006.

Environmental Working Group. "Chemical Families: Mercury Compounds." http://www.ewg.org/chemindex/term/470.

Fialka, J. J. "How Mercury Rules Designed for Safety End Up Polluting." *Wall Street Journal*, April 20, 2008.

Gorbach, S. L. "Antimicrobial Use in Animal Feed: Time to Stop." *New England Journal of Medicine* 345, no. 16 (2001): 1202–1203.

Hauser, R. "Bisphenol A and Female Reproductive Health: Preliminary Results." Lecture, the Department of Community Health and Preventative Medicine Grand Rounds at Mount Sinai Medical Center, New York, NY, June 19, 2009.

‡Lang, I. A., T. S. Galloway, A. Scarlett, W. E. Henley, M. Depledge, R. B. Wallace, and D. Melzer. "Association of Urinary Bisphenol A Concentration with Medical Disorders and Laboratory Abnormalities in Adults." *Journal of the American Medical Association* 300, no. 11 (2008): 1303–1310.

Pollan, Michael. "The Age of Nutritionism: How Scientists Have Ruined the Way We Eat." *New York Times Magazine,* January 28, 2007.

———. "Farmer in Chief: What the Next President Can and Should Do to Remake the Way We Grow and Eat Our Food." *New York Times Magazine,* October 12, 2008.

———. "Mass Natural: With Wal-Mart Going Organic, Where Will Organic Go?" *New York Times Magazine,* June 4, 2006.

———. "Unhappy Meals. Eat Food. Not Too Much. Mostly Plants." *New York Times Magazine,* January 28, 2008.

———. "The Vegetable-Industrial Complex: Bad Spinach that the Government Will Only Make Worse." *New York Times Magazine,* October 15, 2006.

———. "Weed It and Reap." *New York Times.* November 4, 2007.

———. "You Are What You Grow: Will This Year's Farm Bill Make Us Fatter and Sicker?" *New York Times Magazine,* April 22, 2007.

Robinson, Jo. *Pasture Perfect: The Far-Reaching Benefits of Choosing Meat, Eggs, and Dairy Products from Grass-Fed Animals.* Vashon Island, WA: Vashon Island Press, 2004.

Tugend, Alina. "The (Possible) Perils of Being Thirsty While Being Green." *New York Times,* January, 5, 2008.

———. "Teflon Is Great for Politicians, but Is It Safe for Regular People?" *New York Times,* October 14, 2006.

Turtle Island Restoration Network. "Got Mercury?" http://www.gotmercury.org.

U.S. Environmental Protection Agency. "Fish Advisories." http://www.epa.gov/waterscience/fish.

White, D. G., S. Zhao, R. Sudler, S. Ayers, S. Friedman, S. Chen, P. F. McDermott, S. McDermott, D. D. Wagner, and J. Meng. "The Isolation of Antibiotic-Resistant Salmonella from Retail Ground Meats." *New England Journal of Medicine* 345, no. 16 (2001): 1147–1154.

Index